SO-BBB-361

CONSULTATION
with a
CARDIOLOGIST
Coronary
Heart Disease
and
Heart Attack
Prevention

by the same authors
Consultation with a Cardiologist
Coronary Heart Disease and Heart Attack
MANAGEMENT

CONSULTATION
with a
CARDIOLOGIST
Coronary
Heart Disease
and
Heart Attack
Prevention

**Jacob I. Haft, M.D., with
Saretta Berlin**

Nelson-Hall [nh] Chicago

Library of Congress Cataloging in Publication Data

Haft, Jacob, I   1937–
    Consultation with a cardiologist-prevention.

    Includes index.
        1. Heart—Diseases—Prevention. I. Berlin, Saretta,
joint author. II. Title. [DNLM: 1. Heart diseases—
Prevention and control—Popular works. WG113 H139ca]
RC682.H2   616.1′2′05   78–26660
ISBN 0–88229–320–6

Manufactured in the United States of America

10   9   8   7   6   5   4   3   2   1

Contents

Preface

My daily experience with patients is that each office visit leaves an inescapable residue of valid and important questions. Most physicians try very hard to tell their interested patients everything they need to know to beneficially affect the outcome of their particular case. When I tell a patient, for example, that his blood pressure is elevated I deliver what I hope is a complete rationale for his treatment along with the program and medications that I prescribe. And yet, with the best intentions and taking all the time that is possible in the course of a busy office day, I know that many questions remain. As a matter of fact, most of the chapters of this book could quite accurately be called, "What to do *after* the doctor says . . ."

Everyone, myself included, has had the experience of arriving home after a visit to the doctor with questions that did not arise earlier. People who are in good health wonder what they should do to stay that way. Your physician may tell you that everything looks all right and you can assume that you should continue doing whatever it is that is providing you with this nice uneventful history. Questions, however, remain:

"Doctor, I am in pretty good shape now and you tell me that everything is normal, but how do I really prevent a heart attack?

What does a normal electrocardiogram really mean? You tell me that my blood pressure is normal at 130 over 80. What does that mean? Should I take vitamin E?"

Even more important, from the patient's point of view, are those questions that remain after your doctor tells you that he finds something abnormal:

"What is high cholesterol and how do I reduce it? How about triglycerides? I've been a smoker for twenty years; would it help to stop now? Are hypertension and high blood pressure the same? What does a high blood pressure reading mean? What about the reports in the newspaper about cigarette smoking causing heart attacks in young women? Can I drink coffee? How much exercise is good?"

Patients who see the doctor because of specific complaints often come away with a prescription—and a great many unanswered questions:

"How do you know if you're having a heart attack? What is angina? Is it the same as a heart attack? What about chest pains? Which ones do you worry about? Can the electrocardiogram tell if you're having a heart attack?"

These questions are no doubt repeated daily in physicians' offices throughout the world, and a complete answer to each requires some description of the basic physiology and pathology of the heart. Although each question is personal and practical in intent, the conscientious physician recognizes that underlying each one is the basic need to know, "What can I do?" The goal of this book is to answer each of the questions introduced here, and many others, in easily understood and practical terms.

I feel it is vital that physician and patient alike be able to refer to a straightforward, up-to-date, and easily understood compendium of what we know now about heart disease and its prevention. Because I have not been able to find such a book to recommend to my patients, I have attempted to supply the necessary technical material in a form that is easily understood by the concerned layman.

I have endeavored throughout to present a fair picture of heart disease and its current management. Material concerned with its prevention is offered as practically and as completely as is possible, without grinding any well-known medical axes or suggesting nonexistent panaceas. It must be pointed out, however, that agreement among the experts is not yet complete concerning the relative importance or causative power of many of the known risk factors; many questions will be answered fully only when the results of several long-term, large-scale studies become available.

The potential for prevention (the concern of this volume) is great, and most researchers agree that individuals and families at high risk can effectively utilize certain prudent measures suggested by recent findings. Each of the known coronary risk factors is discussed fully. Where disagreement exists it is noted, but in every case sound, practical, and easily followed advice is offered.

Some of the information given here may be objected to by some physicians; others might feel it best that patients not have access to material of this kind. It has been my experience that the contrary is true: the informed patient who is interested enough to pick up a book like this one is almost always benefited by a clear presentation of the facts. I am persuaded, as are many other clinicians working with heart disease victims and their families, that the patient who participates actively in the management of his condition feels better—and in a significant number of cases does better.

The other volume in this series, *Management,* emphasizes the symptoms of coronary disease and their management. Angina Pectoris and heart attack are discussed in detail as *Management* is written mainly for patients who have symptomatic coronary disease. The broader thrust of this volume, *Prevention,* is on risk factor analysis and on ways to ameliorate the risk factors of heart disease.

Aware of the meaning of coronary disease, or concerned with its possible prevention, and cognizant of what can and what cannot be done, the knowledgeable individual can do a great deal to help himself and his family to live a longer, healthier life.

Chapter 1

Heart Disease: The Problem and the Hope

Since the beginning of time, man has known that the heart is his most vital organ—that life itself comes to an end when the heart ceases to beat. As medical science has controlled many of the infectious diseases that have plagued mankind, heart attacks and related cardiovascular diseases have come to be called the twentieth-century epidemic.

Although heart disease is prevalent throughout the world, it appears to be deadlier and more widespread in the so-called advanced nations. Every year in the United States more than one million people suffer a heart attack; more than half of these attacks result in death. Because of this high mortality from heart attacks and other cardiovascular diseases, the United States ranks an almost unbelievable *twenty-fourth* among the world's nations in terms of life expectancy for men. In this country, the toll exacted by diseases of the heart exceeds those of all other causes, including cancer, strokes, and accidents *combined*.

Part of the problem concerning the control of heart disease is the absolute incomprehensibility of these staggering figures: the fact that more than *880,000* people die each year in this country from heart attacks and strokes is probably less meaningful than the young man we used to know who died suddenly at the age of

thirty-five. The cost to American industry of $20 billion is less af-
fecting somehow than the fact that the young man left young children who must somehow be raised and educated in a home suddenly left fatherless.

The statistics describing heart disease patterns throughout the
world are interesting, confounding, and troubling. Since 1956, for
example, the United States has had the world's highest coronary
mortality rate—more people die from heart disease in this country
than anywhere else. But, as other countries "develop," their death
rates from coronary disease begin to approach ours, which has remained fairly constant.

The role of affluence, probably working through its effects
on the customary diet of a nation's people, is underscored by the
fact that during the war, which ended in 1945, and in the years
immediately afterward, the incidence of *myocardial infarction*
(the technical term for a heart attack) throughout Western Europe
was extremely low. In 1948, for example, there were no more than
2,000 deaths due to heart attack in Germany. Compare that to the
figure of 125,000 cardiovascular deaths in the Federal Republic
of (West) Germany in 1970 to get some idea of the tremendous increase in mortality from heart disease in the "developed" areas of
the world.

The same striking increase has also been reported in the
rapidly industrializing areas of Japan, each year showing a tremendous increase in deaths from coronary heart disease over the
year before.

Even the relation to "improved" diet, however, does not account for the wide variety in mortality from heart disease within
countries. Strikingly different mortality rates have been reported
from east and west Finland (which has the highest overall rate in
Europe), north and south Japan, and between different areas of
Italy and Russia. Worldwide statistics, analyzed and collected by
the World Health Organization and others, also indicate increased
mortality from myocardial infarction for men and women of
younger ages.

To the staggering toll of death from heart disease must be
added the significant effect—the cost—of a heart attack to the
family and associates of the victim. Heart disease used to be considered a disease of the elderly; now, for reasons that are not en-

tirely clear, heart attacks, frequently accompanied by sudden or unexpected death, appear to be striking an appallingly large number of relatively young men between the ages of forty and sixty-five. More than a quarter of all heart-related deaths occur in men under the age of sixty-five; half of those disabled by heart disease are under sixty-five years old. Occurring when a man is most important to his wife, his children, his business, and even to his country, this sudden loss of relatively young and productive men either by death or incapacity is an epidemiologic statistic of widespread economic and social importance. It is especially significant that many of the younger people struck down by heart disease tend to be among those who are the more dynamic, more ambitious, and more successful of the population.

Over the past half-century much has been added to our knowledge of the mechanisms and actions of the heart and the many diseases and conditions that affect it. The past twenty years have seen enormous improvements in treatment and diagnostic methods: hospital-based coronary care units to monitor patients with heart attacks, new laboratory tests and treatment techniques, and most recently the development of cardiac surgery to correct problems that underlie some forms of heart disease. With these advances many lives have been saved and many patients previously incapacitated have been returned to active life.

But the impact of these advances on premature sudden death and the occurrence of life-threatening cardiac events has been small. Because more than 50 percent of all deaths from coronary events occur *outside* of the hospital, none of the modern hospital-based wonders of cardiology—pacemakers, intensive care units, or cardiac surgery—can effectively be used to reduce overall mortality from acute myocardial infarction. It is now overwhelmingly clear that only preventive measures, begun early and continued throughout the life of the individual, can achieve any significant reduction in the toll of death and disability exacted by heart disease.

The goal of all preventive medicine is to enable people to die young as late as possible. This means to sail through middle age and into one's later years with unimpaired heart, lungs, brain, and cardiovascular system—a statement that encompasses perhaps all of one's hopes for good health. In terms of heart attack prevention, this is a peculiarly personal drama that is played on a vast impersonal stage where only some of the props are movable: that is, one can bring about healthful changes in one's life *within* the given context of one's unchangeable heredity and resistant environmental conditions.

Studies of large population groups have yielded valuable information concerning the characteristics that are associated with a high incidence of heart disease. Communities studied over long periods of time have revealed that certain factors—inborn traits like diabetes and gout, behavioral characteristics that are manifested as a particular response to stress, social habits like smoking, physical conditions like elevated cholesterol levels, and hypertension—are all associated with an increased incidence of coronary disease. Called *risk factors,* medical shorthand for those circumstances which influence an individual's likelihood of developing disease, such information can be used to predict with some degree of certainty which groups of Americans are at highest risk for the eventual development of heart disease. By understanding which risk factors are present in himself and in his family, and by applying this information to his own lifestyle and physical background, each individual can personally affect his chances of having a heart attack.

Measures undertaken in an effort to reduce one's risk of heart attack have at least two important dividends: each is known to do no harm and there is increasing evidence that their application can have striking benefits of lowering the risk of developing other diseases as well. The cigarettes you give up in an effort to reduce your risk of heart disease, for example, will be of enormous help in keeping you out of the lung cancer and emphysema statistics. There is growing evidence that a diet high in cholesterol and saturated fats may also play a role in the development of some kinds of cancer, so when you begin a lifelong program of low-fat meals you may be embarking on a far-reaching health program. Equally important is the fact that modifying these coronary risk factors is known to do no harm, the first tenet of the Hippocratic Oath.

All of the coronary risk factors have the special quality of being inherently beneficial health measures. Everyone knows the link between stress and stomach problems; when you attempt to reduce the tensions of your life in order to become less prone to a coronary attack, it is helpful to know that you are possibly reducing your risk of stomach ulcers as well. People who exercise sensibly in an effort to modify their risk of heart disease look better, feel better, and respond better—important dividends in anyone's investment program. And the same can certainly be said about the effort to take off weight in order to modify the coronary risk factor of obesity.

Although heart disease is a mass killer, the effort for its control must be made on a particularly personal level. After all the research has been evaluated, it is the individual who must decide, for example, to change his eating habits to reduce his cholesterol levels; each man and woman has to decide for himself/herself whether the coronary risk inherent in heavy smoking is worth it; and each adult must examine his life to determine how it influences the health of his children.

Although a great deal of information concerning coronary risk factors has appeared in the professional literature and in the leading medical journals, unfortunately the research findings that filter down to the popular level have in many cases resulted only in confusion. Even the most careful reader must despair when conflicting studies presented at medical meetings are reported, sometimes inaccurately, in his daily newspaper. Because I feel that information derived from these landmark studies can be used easily and effectively by most individuals to reduce their risk of heart disease, this material is presented in an easily understood, practically applied manner in this book. Aware of his personal risk from factors such as high blood pressure, elevated cholesterol, obesity, stress, and smoking, each individual will hopefully be motivated to alter his way of life, and his family's, toward a more healthful future.

Chapter 2

The Heart
and
How It Works

The heart is a complex and efficient organ with one vital function: to pump blood to all parts of the body. Because it is concerned with the transport of materials to the body's cells, the heart must be understood as the body's prime power source—absolutely essential to the proper functioning of the organism as a whole.

THE BODY'S CELLS

The human body is composed of millions of individual cells. Each has a specific function and purpose, and each is required in some way for the efficient operation of the intact individual. Although these cells are different from each other in many ways—a brain cell differs from a cell in the skin, or from a bone cell, or from a cell in the muscle, gut, or thyroid gland—each of these differently functioning cells has a number of properties in common.

The first of these common properties is that every living cell requires energy to stay alive and to perform its duties. The energy required is produced by a remarkable process called metabolism that goes on within each individual cell using fuel and oxygen supplied to it by the body's circulatory system. The fuels originate from the foods we eat and are usually simple sugars (carbohydrates) or fats. The process of energy production goes on constantly throughout the human body in the tiny subcellular apparatus of each cell. Oxygen, whose presence is critical to most cells, combines with the fuels in a series of chemical reactions to release energy. As the carbohydrates and fats are broken down or "burned," waste products are generated, the most abundant of which is carbon dioxide. Proteins may occasionally be altered to form carbohydrate or fat (usually in the liver), but in most cases they are used only as building blocks to replicate or repair the cells. This production of energy from fuel in the presence of oxygen is called *aerobic metabolism*.

METABOLIC REQUIREMENTS FOR FUEL AND OXYGEN

Cells of different parts of the body vary widely in their requirements for both fuel and oxygen. Skin cells, for example, do not require nearly as much oxygen as do the cells of the brain. This is because cells in the skin are relatively inactive, whereas the cells in the brain are almost always working. This has marked adaptive advantages for human survival in relatively hostile climates. Man can remain in the cold for long periods of time, for example, because circulation to the skin can be reduced almost instantly when needed to conserve the body's heat. When this is done automatically in response to the stimulus of extreme cold, for example, hours may pass before permanent damage to the skin occurs. In contrast, the brain requires the constant delivery of large amounts of oxygen and suffers irreparable damage if its supply is cut off for more than just a few minutes.

The requirements of the metabolic system are such that appropriate amounts of fuel and oxygen must be delivered to actively metabolizing cells as soon as they are needed, and the waste products, especially the carbon dioxide, must be removed promptly. (Waste products that are not removed immediately will poison the cell.) Because many of the body's cells have small amounts of fuel stores, it is the lack of oxygen supply and the failure to remove carbon dioxide that are most critical factors in causing cell damage.

In addition to requiring fuel and oxygen to perform its specific functions, each of the body's cells requires energy to maintain its integrity. That is, it must be able to repair any damage it suffers and in certain situations must be able to replace itself as it ages and dies.

The Blood Vessel System

In order for the cell to live, function, and repair itself, the delivery and removal system must function smoothly and efficiently. In the extraordinary design of the human body, it is the continuously flowing blood conveyed through the vascular system that delivers substances to and from the millions of cells that comprise the organism. Each cell in the body must come in close contact with a branch of the vascular system in order to allow the fuel and oxygen to pass from the blood to the cells and the wastes to go from the cells back into the blood for removal. To accomplish this the blood delivery system is composed of vessels of decreasing sizes.

On the *arterial side,* the system which delivers the oxygen-rich blood to the cells, the main vessel coming from the heart is called the *aorta.* Arteries to the main parts of the body come off the aorta and branch into *arterioles,* or "little" arteries. Beyond these are the smallest branches of the vascular system, the *capillaries,* and it is through the remarkably thin walls of the capillaries that the actual exchange of fuel and oxygen for wastes takes place. Capillaries are as small as 1/100 of a mm in diameter. (The period at the end of this sentence is about ¼ to ½ of a mm.)

After it has been depleted of its oxygen and fuel, the blood picks up carbon dioxide which must be returned to the heart for pumping to the lungs. There it is cleansed of its carbon dioxide and "recharged" with oxygen. The return occurs by way of the *venous side* of the delivery system which, like the arterial side, is composed of vessels of graduated sizes. After the *capillaries,* there are the *venules* or "little" veins, followed by the veins and then the main veins, the *venae cavae,* which drain the whole body and go to the heart.

In this way the blood vessels or blood vascular system operates through the two one-way conduits of the body's circulatory system: the arterial system takes the enriched blood from the heart to the cells and the venous system takes the depleted blood and cellular wastes back to the heart. The blood that returns to the heart by way of the venous system is then pumped by the heart into the lungs through the pulmonary (lung) arteries and arterioles to the pulmonary capillaries which are in close contact to the air we breathe. Here the carbon dioxide is removed and the oxygen is once again picked up by the blood. Waste products other than carbon dioxide are removed by the kidneys and the liver.

Although certain organs of the body, especially the brain and the heart, require a constant supply of oxygen and fuel, there are other parts of the body that have varying needs, requiring large deliveries of blood and oxygen only at certain times. The thigh muscle, for example, requires little fuel or oxygen when it is at rest. If the individual suddenly jump up and begins to run, the thigh muscle must contract and work vigorously; it then requires the rapid delivery of fuel and oxygen and the immediate removal of its waste products. The amount of oxygen and fuel demanded and the blood supply needed to deliver them depend to a large extent on how rapidly metabolism is occurring within the individual cell. By a reflex action which varies the size of the arterioles feeding the area (known technically as *arteriolar dilatation*), the rate of flow of blood can be changed instantly, often to an enormous degree, in response to the needs of a specific part of the body.

Thus whether a constant supply of blood is needed at all times or only at certain times, as when an activated muscle is contracting, the vascular delivery system possesses the ability to supply the appropriate amount of necessary fuel and oxygen almost at once and to promptly remove whatever waste products are present.

THE HEART AS A PUMP

If we consider the type of pump that must be constructed to handle the requirements of this vast and complex vascular system, and if we think for a moment about the materials that are available for the body to work with, then the design of the heart can be seen as eminently rational and very beautiful. The requirements specifically are that there be a constant but varying supply of blood delivering needed fuel and oxygen to the cells of the many different organs of the body. This blood must be moved along, under pressure, through smaller and smaller branches and then be returned to its source. Such a process requires a strong propelling force, a pump, to maintain a head of pressure that keeps the blood moving evenly through gradually narrowing vessels.

This force must also be instantly responsive to the needs of different parts of the body, maintaining the blood pressure fairly evenly while varying the flow as vessels open up (to serve exercising muscles, for example) or close down (when an organ or muscle is at rest and no longer needs an abundant supply). In order for all the cells of the body to receive the fuel and oxygen they require, since only a certain quantity of each can be carried per unit of blood, it is necessary in the normal adult for a total of approximately five liters, or eleven quarts, of blood to circulate per minute through the vascular system at rest.

A pump strong enough to deliver eleven quarts of blood at one stroke would be enormous, much too large to fit in the human body. Consequently the human heart, no larger than a man's fist, is ingeniously designed to contract about seventy times per minute, pumping out about seventy cubic centimeters (about two and one-half ounces) of blood with each stroke, for a total of 4,900 cubic centimeters or just about five liters per minute. In most adults this requires that the heart contract about one hundred thousand times a day. When a person exercises or when he is under stress of any kind, the heart possesses the remarkable ability of increasing its output three- to fourfold to meet the increased demands of the body. This is achieved by increasing the frequency of the pumping action—the *heart rate*—and by increasing the amount of volume put out by each stroke. While the normal heart rate is about seventy beats per minute at rest, the rate can double or almost triple within seconds.

In conditioned skiers, for example, heart rates of over two hundred beats per minute have been recorded just before a big jump. Racing car drivers were recently studied under race conditions using portable electrocardiographic equipment similar to that developed to monitor astronauts on space flights. Drivers' heart rates increased during the course of a stock car race to peaks of almost three times the normal seventy to eighty beats per minute. These maximum rates occurred during exceptional emotional stress, when passing a wrecked car or during a close duel with another racer.

The amount of blood put out by the heart per stroke can go from seventy cubic centimeters (70 cc) per stroke in a normal situation to a volume of two to almost three times that. Under stress, in situations where the cells suddenly require a marked increase in the amount of blood delivered to them, the *cardiac output*, defined as the amount of blood that is pumped per minute, can go as high as twenty liters per minute. The heart's ability to increase the amount of blood it delivers is called the *cardiac reserve,* and the normal heart can call on this capacity to increase its output by a factor of up to four times the normal in response to increased demand.

Diseases of the heart, or diseases of the arteries that feed the heart, can decrease this reserve capacity. With severe abnormalities of the heart a point may be reached where little or no reserve remains. Even a slight increase in demand for cardiac output cannot be met, and patients with these difficulties will experience shortness of breath, considerable weakness, and other symptoms of heart failure.

HOW THE BLOOD DELIVERS

As the main purpose of the cardiovascular system is to deliver fuel and the critically needed oxygen to the cells, a genuine understanding of the work of the heart requires some knowledge of how the blood transports these materials.

The red cells of the blood contain *hemoglobin,* a remarkable substance that has a strong affinity for oxygen. Hemoglobin picks up oxygen where it is present in high concentrations and gives it up where the concentrations are low.

During each circuit that the blood makes through the vascular system it passes through the lungs. As we breathe, air containing oxygen is taken into the lungs. Since the lungs are composed of many small membranes, making up countless tiny air sacs, a large surface area is available for the exchange of gases. Every portion of this extensive membrane system is supplied with thin-walled capillaries that allow the blood to come close to the air that is breathed. Because its concentration is high, oxygen passes easily from the air through the fine lung membranes and capillary walls into the blood where it is picked up by the hemoglobin of the red cells. The lungs are also the site where the waste carbon dioxide, picked up from the cells, crosses from the blood into the sacs to be breathed out.

The blood, now rich with oxygen-laden hemoglobin and depleted of its carbon dioxide, is then pumped to the cells where the oxygen concentration is low. The oxygen is immediately transferred from the red cells to the body cells through the thin walls of the capillaries that come in close proximity to each of the individual cells of the body; carbon dioxide, which is in high concentration at the cellular level, is picked up to be returned to the lungs. Because all of the blood that is eventually delivered to the body cells must be high in oxygen and low in carbon dioxide, it is necessary that all of the blood pass through the capillary system of the lungs.

The heart provides the pumping power to get the blood to the cells of the body and to the capillaries of the lungs. These two pumping operations, however, must be kept separate so that only oxygenated blood is pumped to the cells and only unoxygenated blood to the lungs. This is accomplished neatly by having two separate pumping systems comprise the human heart: the right heart accepts nonoxygenated blood from the veins and pumps it into the lungs, and the left heart takes the oxygenated blood from the lungs and pumps it through the systemic circulation to the cells of the body.

THE ANATOMY OF THE HEART: VALVES

Although separated functionally, the two pumps are anatomically in close apposition to each other and together comprise what we call the heart. Each of the two pumps is made up of a major pump, called the *ventricle,* and a minor or priming pump, called the *atrium,* which delivers the blood from the veins or the pulmonary lung circuit to the ventricles. The right atrium takes the venous blood from the body and acts as a priming pump to deliver the blood to the right ventricle, which then pumps it to the lungs; the left atrium takes the blood from the lungs and acts as a priming pump to deliver the blood to the left ventricle, which then pumps it out to the body.

Between the atria and the ventricles, and between the pump and the major vessels going either to the lungs or to the body, there are important *valves.* This system of valves between the major chambers of the heart and between the heart and the main vessels insures that the blood goes in only one direction; that is, from the veins to the heart to be pumped out through the arteries. Without these fine, filamentous fibrous valves, contraction of the ventricles would force blood backward into the veins and not forward into the arteries as is required for the heart's efficient operation. The valves between the ventricles and the great vessels keep the blood from leaking backward between contractions and serve to insure that the blood always flows forward.

There are two valves on each side of the heart. The *tricuspid valve* lies between the right atrium and the right ventricle and insures that venous blood meant for the right heart is not pumped back into the veins. The *pulmonic valve,* which sits between the right ventricle and the main artery to the lungs, acts to keep the blood which has been pumped into the lungs by the right ventricle from leaking backward into the right heart.

On the left side of the heart the *mitral valve* separates the left atrium from the left ventricle and keeps the blood coming from the lungs from being passed back into the pulmonary or lung veins during contraction of the left ventricle. Between the left ventricle and the aorta, the main artery into which it pumps, the aortic valve keeps the blood which has been delivered into the systemic circulation from leaking back into the left ventricle.

The heart cannot work efficiently unless all of these valves are competent. They must be able to open enough so that they present no obstruction to forward flow and they must be able to close tightly enough so that the blood does not leak backward. Certain diseases, especially rheumatic fever, can cause serious damage to these valves. The primary reason for the vigorous treatment of "strep throat" during childhood is to avoid this possible complication of streptococcal infection.

THE CONTRACTION OF THE HEART

The pumping action of the heart is accomplished by contraction of the heart muscle; mechanically, the contraction rapidly decreases the size of the heart chambers and the blood is squeezed out. The thickness of the muscle in the four chambers of the heart varies and is related to the level of pressure that the chamber must generate. Thus the thickest walled chamber of the heart is the left ventricle because this part of the heart must generate the systemic blood pressure. If hypertension or high blood pressure is present, these walls become even thicker. The right ventricle pumps venous blood to the lungs, an area of low resistance where the pressure is only approximately a fifth of the systemic circulation, so its walls are thinner. (With disease of the lungs, pulmonary hypertension may occur and the walls of the right ventricle will thicken. In this way lung disease can present a hazard to the efficient operation of the cardiovascular system.) The atria, which act only as priming pumps for the ventricles, normally generate only small levels of pressure and hence are thin-walled.

Because of its large number of working muscle cells, the heart itself requires a supply of fuel and oxygen to function, just like other cells of the body. Because the walls of the heart are too thick to allow sufficient nutrients for its needs to be extracted from the blood which it pumps, the heart must have its own blood supply. The arteries which supply the heart are called the *coronary arteries* and they originate as the first arterial branches of the aorta, just as it comes from the left ventricle. There is both a left and a right coronary artery.

Like other arterial beds the coronary arteries branch into small arterioles and then into capillaries, and in this way they feed the muscle tissue of the heart with the oxygen, nutrients, and fuel that it needs. Because the heart works constantly a continuous supply of oxygen and fuel is needed. Although a small amount of fuel is stored in the heart, the need for oxygen is critical and it must be delivered constantly.

Because most of the work of the heart is performed by the left ventricle, the walls of this chamber receive most of the coronary blood flow. If there is an occlusion or narrowing of the artery that feeds a part of the heart, the area deprived of blood will be endangered. When a part of the heart is starved for oxygen, it will first cease to function and then, after a period of time, will suffer permanent damage. When this sequence of events occurs, and a part of the heart muscle is damaged, a myocardial infarction or heart attack has taken place. Because most of the coronary blood flow is needed by the left ventricle, this is the part of the heart most often damaged by heart attacks. How and why heart attacks occur are discussed at length in the next chapter, "The Heart and How It Gets Sick."

HEARTBEAT

An intriguing and critical aspect of the function of the normal heart is the physiology of that awesome occurrence, the heartbeat. The heart beats on its own, automatically, in a regular rhythm that responds to the body's needs by either accelerating or slowing down its rate, or by adjusting the volume pumped out by each stroke. Rather intricate research spanning the last 100 years has revealed that, in addition to its contracting muscle cells and specialized fibrous tissue such as valves, the heart has certain characteristic cells that are similar to muscle but act differently. These specialized cells have the property of automaticity, and can act as pacemaker cells; it is their function to initiate the heartbeat.

The major pacemaker area, normally in control of the heartbeat, is located in the right atrium at the area of the entrance of the main vein that comes from the top of the body, the superior vena cava. This area of specialized tissue is called the *sinus node*. Another area of similarly specialized cells, called the *atrioventricular node* (usually shortened to *AV node*), is located in the part of the right atrium where the main vein draining the lower part of the body enters. This is a subsidiary pacemaker; if the sinus node fails for any reason, the AV node region will take over control of the heartbeat.

Throughout the ventricles there are other potential pacemaker cells. These cells, called *Purkinje cells* after the Bohemian anatomist who first described them, are found in the conduction system and, although quiescent in the normal heart, will take over initiation of the heartbeat if both the sinus and AV node areas fail, or if there is a complete heart block between the atria and the ventricles. In this way the heart is protected by a remarkable series of built-in, standby pacemakers that insure that failure of function or disease in one area will not lead to cessation of the heartbeat and death.

Each of the pacemaker areas has its own normal intrinsic rate; the sinus node is faster than the AV node, and the automatic cells in the AV node area are faster than the ventricular Purkinje cells. Since the functioning pacemaker with the fastest beat controls the heart, it is usually the sinus node that governs the heartbeat. In abnormal circumstances, occasionally a subsidiary pacemaker such as the AV nodal area or a ventricular Purkinje cell will accelerate inappropriately and take over control of the heart, producing rhythm disturbances called *arrhythmias*. Such abnormal rhythms can occasionally lead to severe malfunction of the heart and cause serious consequences to the patient.

THE CONDUCTION SYSTEM OF THE HEART

The heart normally contracts in an ordered and efficient sequence as a result of communication apparatus within the heart called the *conduction system*. Normally the heartbeat originates in the sinus node, as an electrical impulse, and is conducted to the atrial muscle fibers. Shortly after the impulse reaches the atrial muscle cells, the atria contract. The impulse is then conducted from the sinus node of the AV node. The AV node forms the junction between the atrial part of the cardiac conduction system and the ventricular part of the conduction system. After a short delay the impulse is conducted into the specialized intraventricular conduction system (composed of Purkinje cells) and thence to the ventricular muscle cells.

The first part of the ventricular conduction system is a cable of Purkinje cells, called the Bundle of His after the German anatomist who first described it. It divides into two branches, the right and the left bundle branches, going to the right and left ventricles, respectively. Other branches coming off these bundles reach into all parts of the ventricular muscle cells and insure that each of the heart's muscle cells receives the impulse promptly. When the proper sequence of contraction occurs, the blood is squeezed from the heart rapidly and efficiently by the contraction of the heart walls.

HEART BLOCK

The conduction sequence from the sinus node results first in the contraction of the atrium and the priming of the ventricles. After a short delay, caused by a momentary lag in conduction in the AV node, the ventricles contract. Blockage of conduction at any point in the conduction system results in an altered contraction sequence. If conduction is compromised between the atria and the ventricles (atrioventricular block), the pump-priming function of the atria may be lost, and if the blockage is complete there will be no relation between atrial and ventricular contraction and the heart rate will drop. When blockage occurs within the ventricle or in the bundle branches, either right or left bundle branch block may occur. Some of these occurrences have serious effects on the efficiency of the heart, such as complete atrioventricular block, while others, such as right or left bundle branch block, are readily compensated for by the normal heart and have little functional effect.

ELECTROPHYSIOLOGY OF THE HEART CELLS

Electrical events play an important part in heart function, and an analogy can be made between the conduction system of the heart and electrical wires. The individual muscle cells of the heart and the conduction fibers of the heart at rest have a difference in charge or voltage across their membranes. The inside of the cell wall has a negative electric charge while the outside is positive. When the cell is stimulated to depolarize, or if it depolarizes spontaneously, the cell loses this charge and for a few milliseconds becomes nonpolarized; that is, there is momentarily no difference between the charge on the inside of the cell and that on the outside.

All pacemaker cells have the ability to depolarize spontaneously and they initiate the heartbeat in this way. When depolarization of a cell occurs, a current is set up and the depolarization spreads to all the cells contiguous to or connected with the cell which has been depolarized. In this way the electricity is conducted throughout the heart, similar to the conduction which takes place over electrical wires.

When the working myocardial cells in the walls of the heart are depolarized by branches of the conduction system they are stimulated to contract. It is the electrical event conducted down through the specialized conduction system to the working muscle that initiates the contraction or pumping action of the heart.

The electricity generated by the depolarization of the muscle cells of the heart can be measured from outside the body by use of the electrocardiogram. From the sequence of electrical events displayed graphically on the ECG recording, we can make deductions concerning the condition of the heart. The many uses and methods of interpretation of the electrocardiogram are discussed in Chapter 4.

THE NERVOUS SYSTEM AND ITS EFFECTS ON THE HEART

Various normal physiological events lead to a spontaneous increase or decrease in the heart rate. If a person is frightened, angered, exhilarated, or merely exercising or making love, his heartbeat will step up. When a person is at rest or asleep, however, the heart rate will slow down. These normal physiological changes in the heart rate are governed by the nervous system.

The nervous system is composed of a number of separate sub-systems. One of its most apparent parts is the sensory nervous system, which serves to relay messages from specialized organs such as the eyes, ears, nose, and tongue, thus allowing us to experience the outside world by seeing, hearing, feeling, smelling, and tasting. (These nerve endings are connected to cells in the brain where actual sensory perception takes place.) The motor nervous system takes messages from the brain to the muscles of the body and transmits consciously controlled movements.

A less noticed but equally important part of the nervous system, the autonomic nervous system, works quietly and efficiently to maintain the integrity of the body. The autonomic nervous system differs from the sensory and motor systems in that there is no voluntary control, no direct sensory appreciation, and no voluntary motor ability. Automatic and for the most part unconscious, the autonomic nervous system functions quietly to maintain the integrity of the body and control the proper functioning of its important vegetative processes.

When a person is asleep after a big meal, for instance, the autonomic nervous system directs the stomach to churn and move the food so that it can be digested and absorbed. The autonomic nervous system regulates the heart to beat at the needed rate and constricts the vessels to the skin to limit the loss of vital heat if an individual must exist in the cold. It maintains breathing at a rate that provides as much oxygen as is needed and directs the removal of as much carbon dioxide as is produced. The important thing about the autonomic nervous system is that it does all these things, and more, without any conscious direction from the individual.

The autonomic system also comes into play if a person is threatened and must suddenly respond with "flight or fight." In a dramatic situation of fear, attack, or anger, more blood is needed by the muscles in order to respond to the threat. The heart rate will increase to step up the supply of blood and an increased supply of oxygen and fuel will be sent to the parts of the body that need them. All of these factors are mediated by the remarkably responsive autonomic nervous system with no further conscious intervention from the individual.

In order to respond to the body's needs so quickly, the autonomic nervous system is divided functionally and anatomically into two parts, the sympathetic and the parasympathetic nervous systems. The sympathetic nervous system is the dramatic system, coming into play when the body must mobilize its own defenses to deal with stress, either internal or external. The responses of the sympathetic nervous system are an increased heart rate, arousal of the senses, and a feeling of sudden wakefulness and strength—everything the individual needs to fight or to flee. These responses are mediated by the *adrenalin* and *noradrenalin* released from the nerve endings and from the *adrenal gland*.

Adrenalin and noradrenalin prepare the body to defend itself, either by fighting or running, following stimulation of the sympathetic nervous system. The system will respond to emergency situations that are either physical or psychic. The surge of feeling that we get when we are angry or upset, or when we are under physical stress of any kind, is for the most part produced by the sympathetic nervous system.

The parasympathetic nervous system plays a converse role, and keeps the vegetative or maintenance system of the body going. When there is no emergency situation, no stress, and no need for arousal of the sympathetic nervous system—when the body perceives no threats—the parasympathetic nervous system is in control. It acts as the civil servant of the body, performing routine chores that keep the organism going. Parasympathetic nerve endings make sure that the food we eat is absorbed, that the cells of the body receive the blood and oxygen they require, and that the body economy is maintained quietly and efficiently when the organism is at rest or asleep.

These two systems are to some extent antagonistic. There are good arguments to suggest that, once the sympathetic nervous system is involved in the human drama, the parasympathetic nervous system shuts off.

Only when the sympathetic nervous system completes its tasks and ceases its function does the parasympathetic system again come into play. For example, if an executive returns to his office after a big lunch and is greeted by a crisis, the proper response is to first become upset and then defensive and corrective. The parasympathetic nervous system shuts down and the sympathetic nervous system goes to work, preparing to fight the threat posed by the crisis. The supply of blood to the gut is diminished and an augmented supply is sent to parts of the body, such as the brain and certain muscles, which might be needed to counter the threat. Under the circumstances indigestion may follow the big lunch.

If on the other hand the executive returns after his meal to an office where everything is going well, where his secretary is, as usual, doing most of the work, he will relax and digest his meal easily. Perceiving no threats, the parasympathetic nervous system will take over, supplying the gut with what it needs to digest lunch. But if an emergency should arise the sympathetic nervous system will supersede its quieter counterpart and effectively halt the parasympathetic nervous system function.

AUTONOMIC NERVOUS SYSTEM EFFECTS ON THE HEART

The parasympathetic nervous system plays an important role in slowing down the heart when a rapid rate or increased output is not needed. In some few abnormal situations, the parasympathetic nervous system may overreact and lead to inappropriately slow rates. This type of abnormal parasympathetic function can cause heart block.

The sympathetic nervous system, however, has the more important effects on the heart. By way of its chemical mediators, adrenalin and noradrenalin, the sympathetic nervous system accelerates the heart rate, raises the blood pressure, and increases the strength of contraction of the working heart muscle cells. Action of the sympathetic nervous system can also increase the rapidity of conduction from the atria to the ventricles.

These responses were important for primitive man for his survival. If he needed to run or to fight, the parts of his body he needed to defend himself—the muscles and the brain—rapidly received the increased supply of oxygen and fuel required for survival itself. The heart pumped faster and within seconds of his perception of a threatening situation the accelerated blood flow was on its way for the body's defense.

But the sympathetic nervous system can overreact on occasion. Although modern man is rarely faced with the overwhelming physical stress that threatened his primitive ancestors, his sympathetic response to emotional stress is similar and can lead to repeated inappropriate, unnecessary, and possibly damaging sympathetic activity. Sympathetic activation itself causes a strain on the heart and may play a role in stress-related conditions such as angina pectoris and hypertension.

Occasionally, of course, there are illnesses and conditions that require the manipulation of certain nervous system effects. In the armamentarium of drugs available to treat systemic illness in man there are drugs which act like the sympathetic or parasympathetic nervous system. Sympathetic-type drugs are used to accelerate the heart and raise the blood pressure; parasympathetic-type drugs are used to stimulate the vegetative functions, being given after childbirth for example, to help the bladder to empty.

There are also drugs that act to block the effects of either the parasympathetic or sympathetic nervous system when stimulation would be inappropriate. Parasympathetic blockers can be used to raise the heart rate and to decrease gastrointestinal motility. Sympathetic blockers are used to slow the heart rate, lower the blood pressure, and in some instances to treat rhythm disturbances and angina pectoris.

Chapter 3

The Heart and How It Gets Sick: Atherosclerosis and Coronary Artery Disease

In the course of one fairly busy day in the office, I decided to conduct an informal experiment of my own to test how well informed some of the patients were who had been referred to me. My concern with the prevention of heart disease has led me—I am certain of this—to stress education and to insist that my patients know as much about their conditions as I can impart to them.

Most of the people I saw in consultation on that particular day had had heart attacks or angina and were being seen for evaluation of the severity of their conditions.

"Have you ever had coronary artery disease?" I asked in a rather perfunctory tone while taking their case history.

"No, never," was the answer given by many of my patients that day.

"I had a heart attack, Doc, but no coronary artery disease," said one man whose disease process involved almost all of the vessels feeding the heart muscle.

"Coronary artery disease?" said one peppery little woman in tones of disbelief. "Don't I have enough problems with a bad heart?"

When my question took the form, "Have you ever had atherosclerosis?", the answers were not very different. More patients appeared to have heard of atherosclerosis—everyone knew of "hardening of the arteries"—but few appeared to connect it either to coronary artery disease in general or to their heart attacks specifically.

I was astonished, and chastened, to learn that almost none of the patients knew that it was widespread disease of their coronary arteries—usually caused by atherosclerotic deposits—that led to their heart attacks. The fact is that coronary artery disease is the overwhelming cause of most heart attacks, many strokes, and some cases of kidney failure. While it is commonly stated that heart attacks are the number one killer in the United States, what is actually meant is that underlying coronary artery disease is responsible for more cardiovascular and related deaths than any other cause.

Having learned a great deal from these patients during this experiment in communications, I began to wonder whether this striking gap in understanding might have something to do with our failure to control today's epidemic of heart disease, especially of young men.

Would it help, I wondered, if people knew that atherosclerosis has been observed clogging the arteries of children and young adults? That "hardening of the arteries" is not only a disease of the elderly but it also appears to occur in younger people each generation? Does it frighten people too much to know that coronary artery disease produces almost no symptoms in its early stages, and that by the time it signals its presence, usually by cutting off the blood supply to the heart or the brain, it is usually too late to do anything more than retard its progression? (Even more chilling is the fact that all too often sudden death is "the first symptom" of atherosclerosis in the coronary arteries.)

Diseases of the heart and blood vessels kill more than one million Americans per year—an average of two per minute. This high death rate is not inevitable, and life expectancy in the country would gain an impressive eleven years if heart and blood vessel diseases were eliminated.

Atherosclerosis has been described as the killer nobody knows. I feel strongly that shedding some light on its causes and mechanisms of action can go a long way toward its eventual control. For this reason I shall describe in detail exactly what happens in the body in the course of a heart attack; detailed information concerning the *symptoms* of a heart attack are given in the second volume of this series, *Management*.

THE PATHOPHYSIOLOGY OF HEART ATTACKS

Any description of the heart's anatomy and function must conclude that the heart is the keystone of an efficient, beautifully designed, and ingeniously controlled mechanism. The healthy heart functions ceaselessly to pump blood through the body, carrying fuel and oxygen on demand to the cells. It has the remarkable ability of delivering up to four times its normal output, when needed, to continually supply the miles of vasculature of the body with exactly the nourishment needed. For purposes of self-preservation and protection the heart is cradled in the chest behind a strong bone wall of rib and cartilage. Through centuries of development and adaptation the heart has evolved as a strong, well-designed, and well-protected pump. What then can go wrong? How does a heart become damaged? What *happens* in a heart attack?

Although all of the afflictions of man—viruses, bacterial infections, tumors, hormonal abnormalities such as hypothyroidism, and trauma—can affect the heart, its unique anatomy and physiology render it especially prone to specific insults. The valves, for example can develop abnormalities that interfere with their function by impeding blood or allowing it to go in the wrong direction; in many cases valvular problems can be surgically corrected. Abnormal communications between the right- and left-sided chambers of the heart are most often due to abnormal development prior to birth (congenital heart disease) and in many cases can also be resolved surgically.

But the major weakness of the system, and the factor underlying the development of heart attacks, is that the heart is a muscle. Like any other muscle of the body the heart needs immediate oxygen and fuel delivery in order to function; unlike other muscles, however, this need is constant and must be supplied without interruption to sustain life. The heart muscle is thick and, although all of the body's blood must pass through its chambers, there is only minimal diffusion of oxygen and fuel from the blood within the heart into its muscular walls.

As a result, in order to insure a constant supply of oxygen

and nutrients to each muscle cell in its wall, the heart has its own vascular system with arteries (the coronary arteries), capillaries, and veins. The coronary arteries originate in the aorta as the first branches of this great vessel. Oxygenated blood pumped by the left ventricle into the aorta courses through both the right and left coronary arteries to nourish the cells of the heart with the oxygen and food it needs to function and maintain its integrity.

The arteries to the heart muscle are of interest because they are unlike arteries to other parts of the body in two notable ways. First, they act to some extent as end arteries; this means that each area of the heart is supplied only by its own artery. If for some reason this artery is unable to nourish its section of the heart, there is no other artery that can supply blood to that area. The heart does have some capacity to develop vessels from one end arterial bed to another; that is, from a part of the muscle fed by one specific artery to a part normally fed by another. Called *collateral circulation,* this ability to form additional vessels is rudimentary, and except in rather rare instances the collaterals are not sufficient to maintain the normal function of the part of the heart muscle not supplied by its usual artery.

Second, the heart muscle has an area between the outside and inside of the wall that acts as if it were a *syncytium.* A syncytium is defined as an area of cells that are not fed by capillaries but are bathed in blood. This syncytial area between the inside and the outside of the heart allows new arteries to be implanted in the heart muscle and enables them to act as feeder arteries to the heart. This is of importance in the Vineberg procedure, one of the early surgical treatments of coronary artery disease. The cells of the heart muscle also have a system of veins which drain into the coronary sinus and from there to the right side of the heart.

Just like other cells of the body, if the heart muscle cells do not receive sufficient blood supply they will first cease to function; then they become damaged and die, and the process of necrosis or degeneration begins. The heart, as remarkable a muscle that it is, is thus almost totally dependent on its arteries. Coronary artery disease—the clogging of these vital feeder arteries, usually by atherosclerosis—is the condition which underlies most heart attacks.

How the Heart is Damaged by a Heart Attack

A heart attack, also known as a coronary thrombosis, a coronary occlusion, or a myocardial infarction, occurs when the blood supply to part of the heart is impaired. It is initiated by the acute occlusion or closing off of an area of a coronary artery, almost always in a part that has been narrowed by preexisting atherosclerosis. When the blood supply is halted, the area of the myocardium usually fed by that artery becomes *anoxic,* or starved for the oxygen it requires. *Ischemia,* or lack of oxygen and nutrients, activates nerve endings in the heart to signal the severe chest pain of angina or a heart attack. Within minutes the area of the muscle fed by the occluded artery becomes quiescent and stops contracting. If coronary flow to such a starved area of the myocardium is not restored rapidly, the pain persists, and over a few hours irreparable damage to that part of the heart occurs.

Almost immediately after the initial cessation of blood flow, the myocardial cells begin to lose some of their normal components. As they begin to be damaged, potassium leaks from the cell, causing a decrease in the membrane potential across the cell. When this happens the cell is unable to depolarize and repolarize as it did before it was damaged. After a number of hours the damage to the cell is irreversible, and constituents other than potassium are lost, including some of the enzymes necessary for proper functioning of the cell itself. Laboratory determinations for the presence of these enzymes in the blood are used to pin down the diagnosis of myocardial infarction, especially when other clinical signs are inconclusive.

After a period of time, if the area does not receive enough blood flow from other sources to maintain its cellular integrity, the heart cells die and become completely necrotic. Myocardial muscle cells destroyed in this way are not able to regenerate and cannot be replaced by working muscle cells. As these decomposing cells disappear, they are replaced over a period of weeks by fibrous scar tissue. After a heart attack or myocardial infarction, although the heart "heals" and the patient can resume most normal activities, the part of the myocardial wall that is lost through ischemic necrosis is replaced by scar tissue that is no longer able to contract.

An area of scar tissue caused by a heart attack will persist and in most cases will lead to permanent changes on the patient's electro-cardiogram.

HEART FAILURE

It is a tribute to its sound design that the heart can tolerate the loss of significant amounts of working muscle in this way and still be able to supply the needs of the body. Normally, the heart has the capacity to increase its cardiac output by a factor of three or four. When a heart attack causes the loss of muscle tissue, this cardiac reserve—the ability of the heart to call upon its remaining resources to function—decreases, although except in massive heart attacks enough healthy muscle remains to maintain the integrity of the body at rest. If the heart undergoes one damaging attack after another, as is sometimes the case, more and more heart muscle is lost until there is little or no cardiac reserve remaining. As the heart becomes increasingly unable to supply the needs of the body even upon mild exertion or at rest, the process known as heart failure occurs. (Widely misunderstood, the term *heart failure* refers to a gradual process during which the heart is increasingly unable to maintain the body's circulation; *cardiac arrest* is the name given to a sudden and acute stoppage of the heart.)

At the beginning, running, walking fast or climbing stairs will produce symptoms of shortness of breath; as deterioration advances, the heart can supply only the needs of the body at rest. With further loss of muscle mass, the heart is unable to maintain a sufficient flow of blood for even mild or normal activity. Severe failure ensues when the heart is unable to sustain life; eventually shock and, finally, death occur.

Many other things take place at the time of a heart attack. A progression of interrelated physiologic changes is set into motion by the initial occlusion of the vital artery and the subsequent stoppage of its supply of blood to the heart. Chest pains, sweating, nausea, fainting, rhythm disturbances, heart block, shock, and cardiac arrest are all symptoms or results of the heart's starvation, and all are discussed at length in the second volume of this series.

ANGINA PECTORIS

It should be understood that a heart attack is the extreme event that signals the complete loss of adequate blood supply to an area of the heart and the destruction of those heart muscle cells. At the other end of the spectrum are the completely patent, or open, coronary arteries which permit the full and normal function of the cardiac cells. In between those two extremes is the situation where the coronary arteries are not completely occluded but are sufficiently narrowed by atherosclerosis so that under certain circumstances the heart muscle is unable to obtain the amount of blood it requires. During these periods of insufficient supply, the chest pains known as *angina pectoris* may occur.

In 1768 an observant anatomist named William Heberden described a severe cramplike chest pain: "The seat of it, and the sense of strangling, and anxiety with which it is attended may make it not improperly be called angina pectoris" (Latin: *angina,* "pain"; *pectoris,* "of the chest"). Autopsy investigation of these early patients showed that angina pectoris correlated with narrowed coronary arteries. Since the coining of the Latin term, angina pectoris has been used to describe repeated episodes of pain in patients with coronary disease. Angina pectoris is thus understood as the heart's cry for the blood flow it requires. The pain is a signal from the heart to the rest of the body and the message is clear: either reduce the heart's need for oxygen or increase its supply. The most compelling part of the message of angina pectoris is that, if the heart's needs are not reduced or if the supply of blood and oxygen is not increased, the heart is in danger of undergoing irreparable damage.

THE HEART'S NEED FOR OXYGEN

The main cry of the heart is for oxygen; fuel is also necessary, of course, but for several reasons its supply is not so critical. First, a small reserve supply of fuel is always present in the heart muscle and, second, if there is enough blood flow to supply sufficient oxygen to maintain the integrity of areas of the heart, there will be enough fuel in this amount of blood to keep those areas going. Oxygen deprivation is what damages the heart muscle when the blood supply is inadequate.

In the normal situation the coronary blood flow can increase by about a factor of three. That is, if the heart muscle requires increased blood flow, the normal patent coronary arteries can dilate or open enough to increase the flow by about three times the normal amount. But, if atherosclerosis has led to the clogging of a coronary artery, the most narrowed point will act as a governor. Just as a governor on a car limits its speed, a significant obstruction in the opening or *lumen* of a coronary artery will impede the flow of blood through that artery and limit its flow. *Anoxia,* defined as insufficient oxygen to fill cellular needs, develops and the area of the heart fed by this narrowed coronary artery will first become stimulated to signal pain and will then cease to function. When anoxia occurs in this way there is usually enough blood flow to maintain cellular integrity but it may not be sufficient to allow the heart muscle to contract and function.

This is because most of the oxygen required by the heart is needed for its contractile functions. The amount necessary to maintain cellular integrity or to maintain the resting potential across the membrane is relatively small when compared to the amount of oxygen that is necessary to keep the heart pumping. It is the steady contraction of the heart muscle that requires energy, so oxygen is needed continuously to burn fuel and yield this energy. Although the heart muscle requires a continuous supply of oxygen, the amount it needs varies at different times in relation to the degree of its activity.

First, the number of contractions per minute will have a direct effect on the amount of oxygen consumed. If the heart beats 80 times a minute it requires more oxygen than if it were beating at a rate of 60 to 70 per minute, and at 100 or 120 beats per minute it needs more oxygen per minute than if it were beating at a rate of 80 per minute.

The oxygen requirement is also related to the amount of force that must be generated by the heart; that is, the level of blood pressure that the heart generates. The higher the blood pressure the harder the muscle must contract and the more oxygen it will take for the development of the contraction. Hence if the heart generates a blood pressure of 140 it needs more oxygen than if it were generating a blood pressure of 120, and if it generates a blood pressure of 185 or 200 it will require even more oxygen than it did at 100 or 120 millimeters of mercury. So the second major determinant of oxygen consumption is the blood pressure.

The third determinant of the oxygen requirement is the strength or rapidity of contraction and the velocity and vigor with which the heart contracts. This is normally determined to a large extent by various substances present in the blood that result from the activity of the autonomic nervous system. When adrenalin and noradrenalin are released, the heart is stimulated and contraction occurs more rapidly and with much more vigor than when these nervous system mediators are not present. Sympathetic stimulation thus enhances heart function and increases its need for oxygen. Drugs such as digitalis and glucagon that improve cardiac performance also lead to increased cardiac oxygen consumption.

The length of time spent in contraction of the heart will also determine its oxygen or energy requirement. If the heart spends more time in *systole,* or contraction, and less in *diastole,* or relaxation, there will be an increase in the amount of oxygen that is required. Several factors act to lengthen the time spent in contraction. If there is a narrowing of the aortic valves so that it takes a longer time for each stroke to deliver blood from the ventricle, oxygen consumption is increased. An increase in the heart rate causes relatively more time to be spent working in systole, and hypertension may also lead to a prolongation of each contraction.

The tension developed by the heart also affects its oxygen consumption. Tension relates to both the pressure that must be developed as well as to the radius of the chamber that is contracting. Thus the size of the heart is an important factor; that is, the larger the heart, the greater its requirement for, and utilization of, oxygen.

The Vital Left Ventricle

To summarize, the oxygen requirements of the heart are determined by heart rate, blood pressure, vigor and speed of the contraction, the period of time spent in contraction versus that spent in relaxation, and the size of the heart's ventricular chamber. Because the left ventricle performs most of the work of the heart and is its thickest walled chamber, angina and most of the other effects of coronary artery disease are seen mainly in this most important chamber of the heart. The left ventricle must develop sufficient pressure to drive the blood through the systemic circulation and must be able to contract enough to produce a satisfactory cardiac output. The right ventricle is needed to get the blood into the pulmonary artery but some important experiments have shown that the animal heart can function to some degree without its right ventricle. Some cardiac reserve is lost, but cardiac output and cellular integrity are usually maintained.

The atria are important because their contractions act to prime the pumping ventricles and increase the efficiency of the heart, but their function is not nearly so critical as the left ventricle's. Left ventricular function uses most of the oxygen consumed by the heart, and it is the coronary artery problems involved with the blood supply to the left ventricle that cause the symptoms of angina pectoris and myocardial infarction.

HOW OXYGEN STARVATION DAMAGES THE HEART'S CELLS

Given the constant requirements of the heart for oxygen as well as the factors that increase its needs, it is relatively easy to understand how the cells of the heart can be damaged when one of the arteries feeding it becomes narrowed or occluded by atherosclerosis. Stated concretely, a somewhat compromised artery feeding the heart of an otherwise normal individual whose blood pressure is 130 over 80, whose heart rate is a normal 72, and who is at rest with no excitement, will probably be able to deliver enough blood to the myocardium to avoid symptoms. If the situation suddenly changes and this person must run up the stairs or must respond vigorously to exercise or emotional exertion, he requires an immediate increase in blood flow to his body. His sympathetic nervous system will become activated, increasing his heart rate and blood pressure and causing his heart to contract more vigorously and rapidly. In this way three of the four determinants for the requirement of oxygen and blood flow are increased. If the compromised coronary artery feeding a part of the myocardium is sufficiently narrowed so that blood flow cannot increase, the oxygen supply to the left heart cannot be stepped up. Anoxia, or oxygen starvation, to the heart will develop, signaled by the chest pain of angina pectoris. If the requirements for blood flow are not reduced (by stopping the activities that led to increased demand), ischemic damage to the heart may occur.

Physical exertion—running, climbing stairs, or lifting heavy packages—can lead to angina, as can any event that stimulates sympathetic nervous system activity—stress, anger, or even cigarette smoking.

The medical treatment of angina pectoris is rational and practical, designed to decrease the oxygen need of the heart or to allow increased blood flow to the heart. If an individual experiences angina on exertion he can often control the pain by the simple expedient of resting; the heart rate will slow, the blood pressure will go down, and the sympathetic tone abates. If the arteries allow enough flow, the pain will usually go away in a few minutes. This is most often the case in mild and infrequent angina.

But frequently the individual with severe recurrent angina pectoris cannot reverse the symptoms of pain by rest alone. Drugs that block the cardiac stimulation of the sympathetic nervous system, called beta-blockers, are used in cases of severe pain to decrease the heart rate and lower the blood pressure while at the same time, most importantly, blocking the effects of added sympathetic stimulation. Patients on beta-blocking drugs thus exercise at a lower heart rate and lower blood pressure. In situations involving anger or emotional stress, the beta-blocking drugs spare the patient the full brunt of sympathetic stimulation that would otherwise bombard the heart and cause it to beat faster.

Angina is also controlled in a different fashion by the family of drugs called nitrates that include the familiar nitroglycerin, amyl nitrate, and the longer acting nitrates. These drugs work by relaxing the smooth muscle in the walls of the blood vessels. In this way the peripheral arteries are dilated and the blood pressure is slightly decreased, effecting a reduction in the work load of the heart. Nitrates also dilate the veins and decrease the amount of blood returning to the heart; less blood returning to the heart decreases its size and reduces its requirements for oxygen. And to some extent the nitrates also dilate the coronary arteries and allow them to deliver more blood flow to the heart muscle. Recently, it has been demonstrated that coronary arteries can occasionally actively constrict, narrowing or closing off their lumen. This can happen in arteries that are partially constricted by atherosclerosis or very rarely in coronaries that are normally open. Such constriction can cut off blood flow and may cause angina at rest. The vasodilating effects of the nitrates are effective in reopening these areas of active narrowing. Understanding what determines the demands of the heart for oxygen allows the rational use of a variety of therapeutic modalities for the treatment and prevention of angina pectoris.

ATHEROSCLEROSIS

In most instances, the basic process that underlies the development of coronary artery disease is atherosclerosis, and it is the control of this pervasive clogging of the arteries that comprises the major thrust of heart attack prevention today. To clear up any misunderstanding, it should be understood that the general term *arteriosclerosis* literally means "hardening of the arteries," and is used to refer to any disease that thickens or hardens the arteries. *Atherosclerosis* is the name given to the specific disease of the blood vessels characterized by fatty deposits on the inside of large- and medium-sized arteries. Atherosclerotic deposits in the arteries leading to the heart, brain, and kidneys can cause angina and heart attacks, strokes, and renal failure, respectively.

The atherosclerotic process has been known for centuries, since the beginning of the use of postmortem examination to understand disease. It was noted by early pathologists that patients dying at an advanced age were frequently found to have marked thickening in the walls of their arteries. Patchy areas of raised yellow-white deposits would often be found obstructing the lumen, or opening, of the artery. In some instances this process was observed to narrow the opening of an artery to a pinpoint or to completely occlude it, blocking all blood flow through that artery. In the late nineteenth century it was noted that even young people who died suddenly would be found on postmortem examination to have advanced atherosclerosis of their coronary arteries. Some time later, at the beginning of the twentieth century, the physical symptoms of angina pectoris and myocardial infarction were specifically related to the presence of occlusive atherosclerosis in the coronary vessels. Dr. James B. Herrick, in 1912, first clearly described the criteria for making the diagnosis of coronary atherosclerosis in a living human. Prior to his work the diagnosis could be made with certainty only by postmortem examination.

Atherosclerosis attacks not only the coronary arteries but can also occur in any of the arterial beds of the body. The arteries involved are usually the large- and middle-sized ones and the symptoms are determined by which organ or part of the body is affected when blood flow to them is compromised or impeded by atherosclerosis. A common site of atherosclerosis is in the arteries that go to the legs. When these large major arteries are partially closed by atherosclerosis, the individual may notice first that he cannot exercise strenuously without developing soreness and aching in the calf muscles. The leg pain is usually effective in curtailing the activity to a tolerable level, but if the individual continues to exercise the muscles may cramp, tightening up on their own and causing severe discomfort. Any actively functioning tissue, in this case the exercising calf muscles of the legs, requires increased blood flow to supply more oxygen and fuel and to promptly remove wastes. If the arteries feeding the legs are narrowed by atherosclerosis, the flow can rise only to a certain level and not beyond. If the active muscles need more blood flow than this governor type of situation will allow, ischemia, or starvation, develops and leg cramps will ensue.

Shortly after exercise is halted, the discomfort in the legs is relieved because the need for blood flow decreases to a level that can be supplied through the compromised artery. The development of symptoms of leg pain during exercise that are relieved by rest is called *intermittent claudication,* and it is almost always a sign that the arteries leading to the legs are narrowed by atherosclerosis. As the disease progresses and there is further arterial narrowing, less and less exercise is required to produce ischemia. Early in the disease, for example, the individual may be able to walk at a normal pace without any symptoms, experiencing pain only if he runs or climbs stairs rapidly. As the atherosclerotic process advances, he may find that even walking quickly will produce pain. Eventually walking at a normal pace for progressively shorter distances will become difficult and pain filled. With further progression of the disease pain may develop even at rest; if the vessels continue to narrow, severely compromising blood flow to the skin, ulcers may develop and, if untreated, gangrene may set in, necessitating removal of a toe, a foot, or a leg. The symptoms of intermittent claudication are exacerbated by smoking, and the use of tobacco is absolutely forbidden to patients exhibiting these signs of impaired circulation to the legs.

Although atherosclerosis in the arteries to the legs is usually relentlessly progressive, its development usually takes place over a period of many years. The extreme case that requires amputation is relatively rare. Patients with intermittent claudication can help avoid these consequences by avoiding situations of sympathetic stimulation (including stress and smoking), by avoiding extremes of temperature to their legs, by meticulous foot and leg hygiene, and by the regular use of specific exercises.

Atherosclerosis attacks other vascular beds with the same destructive power. The arteries to the brain are frequently affected. If atherosclerosis results in significant narrowing of these cerebral vessels, especially in older people, aberrations of memory, difficulty with mentation, and periods of dizziness and fainting may occur. In its rapid or acute form, this arteriosclerotic process may lead to strokes. The precipitating factor in the development of a stroke is often an acute occlusion by a blood clot of an already narrowed artery. Stroke and its relationship to atherosclerosis, hypertension and coronary artery disease are further discussed in Chapter 5.

Atherosclerosis can also affect the arteries leading to the kidneys, resulting in renal ischemia and some forms of hypertension.

THE CAUSES OF ATHEROSCLEROSIS

Although the anatomical and physiological effects of atherosclerosis have been recognized for many years, the mechanism of its development and its immediate cause are still under intense investigation and the subject of significant scientific controversy.

Over the years, however, a number of plausible theories based on observations in the experimental and pathological laboratories and on data accumulated from studies of large groups of people have been developed. The application of these theories forms the basis for current measures suggested for the prevention and control of atherosclerosis.

The major thrust of research into the causes of atherosclerosis centers around the relation of cholesterol and lipids in the diet to atherosclerotic heart disease. This relationship was first suggested by the work of two Russian physicians who worked in the early part of this century. Ignatowsky noted that autopsy evidence of arteriosclerosis was present only in men who ate diets rich in animal fat and Anitschkow developed arteriosclerosis in rabbits by feeding them pure cholesterol. (This work is described more fully in Chapter 6.)

Since these early observations, which were remarkable because no one had ever linked diet to the development of atherosclerosis prior to this time, experimental work in laboratories all over the world has confirmed these findings in a variety of experimental animals. Dietary manipulation and in some cases hormonal alteration to produce hypothyroidism have produced atherosclerosis in rats, dogs, cats, chickens, monkeys, and other experimental animals.

CHOLESTEROL AND ATHEROSCLEROSIS

In addition to experimental evidence that feeding high levels of cholesterol, and thus artificially raising the cholesterol levels in the blood, leads to the formation of atherosclerosis, the medical literature contains a myriad of epidemiological studies conducted on humans that link the occurrence of atherosclerosis, especially in the coronary arteries, with high levels of cholesterol and other lipids (fats) in the blood. It has been known for years that individuals with very high cholesterol levels are prone to develop premature coronary atherosclerosis; when families of these patients are studied, the history that emerges is usually dotted with premature heart attacks and early sudden death, especially among its male members. These patients are considered to have primary hypercholesterolemia.

Although the genetic origin of these traits is not entirely worked out, it appears that elevated cholesterol of this type is carried in families as an autosomal recessive trait with varying penetrance. These arcane words mean that the gene carrying this trait is not sex-linked but is expressed by males and females. Since it is a recessive trait, it takes two genes, one from each parent, to produce offspring who are markedly hypercholesterolemic. If only one gene is present, the individual will have either normal or only moderately high cholesterol levels. Since the genes are of varying penetrance, even if they are present the cholesterol level may be normal.

This is a gross oversimplification of the inheritance of the tendency toward an elevated cholesterol level because the genetic patterns are complex and it is not entirely known exactly how the trait is transmitted from one generation to the next. Elevated cholesterol levels do tend to run in families, however, and these families are usually found to have a high incidence of premature death from coronary heart disease.

The Ultrafiltration Process

The mechanism that relates high cholesterol levels in the blood with the development of atherosclerotic plaque is, like so many other things, not completely understood at the present time. One theory holds that during contraction of the heart the blood is pushed against the vessel wall forcefully, causing some of the serum (the clear, fluid part of the blood) to filter through the inside layer of the blood vessel, the *endothelium,* and end up within the vessel wall. All of the constituents of the serum except the lipids are removed from the wall by the body's normal defense mechanisms. The lipids, especially cholesterol, are not so readily removed and may accumulate to form a gradually enlarging atherosclerotic plaque.

This theory of *ultrafiltration* of the serum into the vessel wall fits with the epidemiological findings that patients with hypertension or high blood pressure tend to be more prone to develop coronary disease. With the greater driving force of high blood pressure pushing the serum into the vessel wall, it would be expected that atherosclerosis would be accelerated. Anything which increases the permeability of the endothelium, such as the presence of clots on the inside surface of the blood vessel or the presence of the sympathetic nervous system stimulators, adrenalin and noradrenalin, would also abet the ultrafiltration process and may help to explain the finding that people under chronic stress tend to develop atherosclerosis readily and at a relatively early age.

Another theory of atherosclerosis relates damage to the inside of the blood vessel to the development of cells within the vessel wall (originally muscle cells) that accumulate cholesterol and degenerate into atherosclerotic plaques. All of the circumstances that increase vascular permeability also damage the endothelium and stimulate these muscle cells to take up cholesterol.

Blood Clots

The relationship of coronary atherosclerosis to blood clots, sympathetic nervous system activity, and chronic stress now appears repeatedly in data derived from large epidemiologic studies, and offers a promising direction in cardiac research. The role of atherosclerotic plaque in the precipitation of a heart attack is thought to be due to the gradual narrowing of the artery until blood flow is critically impeded, to a sudden hemorrhage into the blood vessel wall under the atherosclerotic plaque, or to the sudden occlusion of a previously narrowed area of a coronary artery by a blood clot. Blood clots, or *thrombi,* clogging the artery frequently play a central role, but the exact mechanism of why, how, or when a clot forms in an artery is still unsettled and remains a matter for extensive research and investigation.

Blood clotting is a complex process. When a blood vessel is damaged, when you cut your finger for instance, a whole complex of chemical interactions is set into motion to repair this insult to the tissue. *Platelets,* small formed bodies in the blood, will aggregate or stick together to form a plug to stop the bleeding; if this is insufficient, a cascade of interactions takes place that transforms the soluble protein in the blood into the solid form of a *fibrin clot,* apparent on the skin as an ordinary scab.

Within the vasculature, inside the blood vessels themselves, however, it is usually highly inappropriate and dangerous for this kind of clotting to occur. As we have noted many times, the arteries must remain open to nourish the cells of the body and a clot within an artery will narrow the lumen and impede the supply. In situations of inappropriate bleeding, in case of an injury or surgical incision, for example, the formation of a clot is necessary and desirable. But, within the vascular system itself, a clot is a hazardous occurrence.

In the wisdom and economy of the human body there is a system which acts as a safety mechanism to deal with small clots that may form within the bloodstream. An inappropriate clot will activate this system and small clots will be destroyed before they can clog a vessel; in this way the delivery system of the vasculature will remain open. This system is called the *plasmin-plasminogen* system and it operates by destroying the fibrin that holds the clots together.

The clots that form in the slower moving venous system are composed of fibrin and red and white cells. If these clots are not small enough to be destroyed by the quite marvelous and always active plasmin-plasminogen system, the presence of the clots will further irritate the veins, resulting in the disease of venous inflammation called *thrombophlebitis*. The most dangerous aspect of thrombophlebitis, especially when it occurs in the large veins of the legs, is the possibility that a small piece of a clot may break off and travel by way of the venous system into the right side of the heart. From there these dangerous and inappropriate clots may go into one of the lungs, causing a *pulmonary embolus* or lung clot that can be quite serious. In order to avoid these catastrophic events, anticoagulant drugs, which inhibit the formation of fibrin in the vascular system, are used to prevent thrombophlebitis and to retard the development of clots if vein inflammation is already present.

In the arterial system clots usually originate as *platelet emboli;* that is, the platelets that are always present as a safety mechanism to avoid life-threatening bleeding are somehow traumatized to stick together or to aggregate inappropriately. Fibrin joins the platelets and together they develop into a "white clot," one that does not contain red cells. When such a clot lodges in an area of the vasculature that is too narrow to allow its passage, the platelet clot may in some cases pick up red cells and become a typical blood clot. In any event, the platelet clot is currently thought to play a large role in the development of a heart attack. These clots in the arterial system, occluding the coronary arteries usually at a point of previous narrowing, are suspected of leading to acute myocardial infarction or heart attack in many instances.

The role of platelet aggregation in heart attacks is underlined by some important work done in the late 1960s and early 1970s by Dr. John Hampton and his associates at Oxford. These English researchers have shown that patients with heart disease tend to have a greater degree of platelet "stickiness," apparent as a tendency toward aggregation, than do those patients who have no underlying coronary artery disease. Using a variety of platelet tests, these workers have shown that platelets collected from people with coronary artery disease aggregate more easily than platelets collected from normal controls. Because platelets normally have a negative electrical charge, when placed in an electric field they move toward the positive pole. Any increase in speed in this movement toward the positive pole would indicate that the platelets are more negatively charged, and it has been correlated with the observed tendency for platelets to aggregate or stick together. Interestingly, patients with ischemic heart disease show an abnormally rapid movement of platelets within the electrical field. When stimulated with various substances in the laboratory, usually either ADP or noradrenalin, these platelets respond more easily and move more rapidly toward the positive pole than do platelets from people without coronary disease.

These intriguing findings of platelet abnormalities in patients with coronary disease have also been found by many other investigators and raise an important question: is it the platelets themselves that are abnormal in those with heart disease or is it something in the patient's blood serum that causes the platelets to be more sensitive to stimuli that cause aggregation?

An interesting series of experiments suggests that it is some factor in the serum that causes the platelets to move abnormally in the electric field. On sophisticated analysis, this factor has been found to be present in a lipid or fat fraction of the blood that travels with the beta lipoproteins. Since the beta lipoprotein also carries cholesterol, this suggests that the formation of dangerous clots, the presence of coronary artery disease, and the presence of high cholesterol levels in the blood may be linked by way of this substance that correlates with both the propensity of platelets to clot and elevated cholesterol levels. We must note that, although these findings are of great interest to researchers all over the world, the relationship remains on the level of conjecture and a great deal of work remains to be done. The application of these data to clinical medicine may not be practical for some years to come.

Another theory holds that the intravascular platelet clot may also act to initiate the atherosclerotic process. Some investigators have suggested that the presence of a small clot on the inside surface of the vessel wall may injure the epithelial membrane, making it more permeable to the ultrafiltration of serum. This may enhance the deposit of cholesterol on the vessel wall and lead in this way to the development of atherosclerotic plaque.

In recent years, a more central role for platelets in the development of atherosclerosis has been suggested by a number of medical researchers. It has been shown that any damage to the inside (endothelium) of a blood vessel will cause platelets to adhere to the area of damage. In addition to making the endothelium smooth again however, substances released from the platelets enter the vessel wall and stimulate muscle cells deep in the wall to migrate to the area just under the endothelial surface. These muscle cells then take up cholesterol and other lipids from the blood stream and change into foam cells, the precursor of the formation of an atherosclerotic plaque or area of atherosclerosis in the blood vessel. If no repetitive damage to the endothelium occurs, the foam cells may regress without leading to atherosclerosis and may again return to being ordinary vascular muscle cells. But if damage recurs, the repeated stimulation from the platelets may lead to permanent and progressively more severe atherosclerosis of the vessel wall. Thus, the platelets and the part they play in clotting in vessels may be central to the development of atherosclerosis. The fact that all the known coronary risk factors are associated with enhanced platelet activity support the theory. Diabetes, cigarette smoking, high fat diets, and high cholesterol levels all have marked effects on platelet function and on the tendency for platelets to aggregate.

SYMPATHETIC NERVOUS SYSTEM ACTIVITY AND ATHEROSCLEROSIS

Another epidemiological observation that has intrigued and stimulated researchers for years is the well-documented relationship between stress and the development of atherosclerotic heart disease. It is an all too common finding, one of the many tragedies associated with coronary disease, that success-oriented men— dynamic, aggressive, and usually young—are prone to develop premature heart disease. This Type A coronary-prone behavior pattern is discussed in Chapter 7.

Persons with Type A personality characteristics have been found to have both a higher incidence of coronary artery disease and an increased rate of fatal heart attacks. People who are the opposite, called Type B personality, have little of this aggressive drive and show certain interesting biological differences. By laboratory analysis, for example, Type A personalities tend to have more rapid blood clotting, higher cholesterol levels, and increased excretion of the substances know as *catecholamines*—adrenalin, noradrenalin, and their breakdown products, all of these being, of course, factors associated with the development of heart disease.

The release of substances known as *catecholamines* is especially significant. As noted in the section on normal cardiac physiology, the sympathetic nervous system is activated during stress and substances known as adrenalin and noradrenalin are released. This catecholamine response is an important reaction to stress because it supplies the extra burst of strength and energy that is needed in a sudden emergency. This ability to quickly mobilize his energies enabled prehistoric man to survive his hostile environment.

Modern man also requires the assistance of sympathetic catecholamine effects when he finds himself in a truly threatening emergency situation. With the help of a catecholamine burst people under severe stress are occasionally able to perform truly impossible tasks; the mother who can lift a car to free a child pinned under its wheels is operating with the added strength supplied by the sympathetic nervous system. The catecholamines are powerful aids that make the body more efficient and better able to deal with unusual stress.

Modern living, however, is filled with frustrations, and adults who function today are subject to all kinds of stress. Although these conditions are not of the same order as the predators that threatened prehistoric man, they appear to elicit the same kind of sympathetic response, especially marked in individuals with Type A coronary-prone personality characteristics. These people respond to even minor stress with marked stimulation of the sympathetic nervous system and the subsequent release of large amounts of catecholamines. Continuously high levels of sympathetic activity called up in this way may do considerably more harm than good. That is, the same flow of catecholamines needed to fight a saber-toothed tiger is clearly an inappropriate response to the almost constant modern stress of traffic jams, noisy crowded streets, and the strain of staying afloat in spite of increasing financial demands. Thus, while the catecholamine response is necessary and beneficial in certain emergency situations, in many cases it is called up unconsciously when there is no proper outlet for it. It also appears that the coronary-prone Type A individual overreacts to stress of all kinds and responds with a large catecholamine release to situations that the noncoronary personality would judge to be merely difficult.

The benefits of catecholamine stimulation—the energy and strength it provides—must, like everything else in this world, be paid for. In cardiovascular terms, the system is taxed in several ways to provide this increased strength. There is first an increase in heart rate and blood pressure, as well as an increase in the strength of contraction of the heart. With this increased heart rate, people under sympathetic stimulation may also have an increase in the irritability of the heart, a problem in individuals with prior history of heart trouble since it may lead to disturbances in the heart's rhythm. With sufficient catecholamine stimulation, the blood pressure can rise to such an extent that an artery in the head may bleed, causing a stroke.

As far back in lipid research as Anitschkow, it was observed that animals injected daily with sympathetic catecholamines while on a high cholesterol diet developed more severe and widespread atherosclerosis than animals subjected to a high cholesterol diet alone. The definitive explanation of this link between the catecholamines and atherosclerosis remains relatively unsettled, although there are a number of sympathetic nervous system effects that could possibly be related to the development of atherosclerotic plaque. For example, catecholamines cause an increase in blood pressure in addition to increasing both heart rate and cardiac output; the stepped-up blood pressure may facilitate the ultrafiltration of serum and cholesterol into the vessel walls.

In addition, it has been known for years that adrenalin and noradrenalin cause the blood to clot more rapidly than it would otherwise. Teleologically—that wonderful word that means directed toward a purpose or useful end—this is an extremely beneficial effect; if a man is going into battle or if he is threatened by serious physical injury, rapid clotting has great survival value. Without this sympathetic catecholamine effect, probably mediated by way of the platelets, any injury might cause life-threatening blood loss.

But an inappropriate increase in the tendency of the blood to clot may be dangerous. As we have noted, clotting within the vascular system is an extremely undesirable situation that can cause serious problems throughout the cardiovascular system. Since catecholamines are potent platelet aggregating agents, it is easily understood how they can readily lead to hazardous clotting. Also noteworthy is the fact that patients who are known to have coronary artery disease respond more readily and more vigorously to catecholamine stimulation; in laboratory analyses, their platelets are shown to aggregate more vigorously than do those of normal patients.

Depending on which theory of atherosclerotic formation is operant, an intravascular clot induced by catecholamine stimulation may itself stimulate the formation of an atherosclerotic plaque, or the presence of the clot may make the vessel wall beneath the clot more permeable to ultrafiltration of serum. Either way the formation of an intravascular clot caused by catecholamine response may be the genesis of arterial clogging. Animal studies have shown that sympathetic stimulation and stress can cause platelet aggregation within the vessels of the heart. If atherosclerosis is related in this way to the formation of inappropriate intravascular clots, the biochemical or physiological link between stress and atherosclerotic heart disease may be via the catecholamines secreted in excess during stress which cause the platelets to clot on the inside walls of the arteries.

A great deal of research remains to be done, but this appears to be an important clue to the question of why people who perceive themselves to be under stress most of the time show both increased atherosclerosis and increased incidence of heart attacks.

Chapter 4

How to Estimate Your Risk of Heart Attack: Risk Factor Analysis and Your Coronary Profile

In the last twenty years remarkable and important advances have been made in the identification of coronary risk factors—those physical, biochemical, or social characteristics known to be associated with a high risk of heart disease. Formerly known mainly to physicians and health professionals, terms like "high cholesterol" and "hypertension" are now only too familiar to a frequently confused public. And yet, the only possible hope for the prevention of heart attacks lies in the *individual* application of this kind of health information.

As a result of studies of large populations like that in Framingham, Massachusetts, and elsewhere, we now know a great deal about the factors which predispose people to coronary disease and heart attacks. Combined with laboratory studies detailing the biochemistry of the disease and clinical studies of both human and animal subjects, these findings enable us to say with some certainty that high blood pressure, high cholesterol levels, and cigarette smoking are associated with increased risk of heart disease. Factors like obesity and a low level of exercise are also implicated, as are heredity and the individual's response to stress.

But the important matter of using this rough epidemiologic road map to chart your individual risk of heart attack is not quite so simply done. The problem is that statistics apply only to large groups of people or populations; their application on the individual level is still highly uncertain. Statistically, the results of a large study like that done in Framingham only tell us that over the twenty-year period of the investigation, when a group of people with a high incidence of the various risk factors was compared with a group where the factors were not present or present at very low levels, the rate of heart disease was significantly greater among the former group. This does not mean, for instance, that everyone with high cholesterol had, or will have, a heart attack; it does suggest, however, that their risk is much greater when compared to people with low cholesterol levels.

But the statistics regarding coronary risk factors are helpful in at least two respects. When we know the characteristics that are associated with an increased risk of heart attack we can take measures aimed at modifying these coronary risk factors. And these measures have an added utility in that they are known to do no harm and may in fact be of benefit in the prevention of other diseases as well. Risk factor analysis suggests that the control of elements like smoking, high blood pressure, cholesterol levels, and the like may indeed significantly alter our tendency toward heart disease. Although the beneficial results of modifying the coronary risk factors are not yet fully proven, it is reasonable to expect that efforts toward this end will pay off in terms of improved health.

In addition to reducing coronary risk, people can derive other health benefits from changing habits or treating abnormalities that may predispose them to heart attacks. Cigarette smoking, for example, plays a role in several other serious diseases—lung cancer and emphysema among them. High blood pressure has been clearly implicated as a precipitating factor in strokes as well as in coronary heart disease, and obesity, in addition to placing an extra strain on the heart, is both uncomfortable and unfashionable.

KNOW YOUR RISK FACTORS

Since it is clear that modifying most coronary risk factors will do no harm and may prove extremely beneficial in improving general health and well-being, how does one go about it?

The best place to begin is in your doctor's office. And the best time to begin is when you are feeling well. Prevention is the goal;

heart attacks happen, of course, but it is just good sense to apply every means known in a sound effort to avoid an acute event.

Every man over forty should see his doctor at least once a year in the absence of symptoms. If he is not feeling well, or if he has an underlying condition of some significance, the appointments should be more closely spaced. Men with a family history of premature death from heart disease would do well to begin to see a physician earlier in adulthood, during their late twenties or early thirties.

For women the situation is slightly different. The incidence of coronary heart disease is usually quite low among younger women, although after menopause this incidence increases rapidly. A strong family history of premature cardiac death or disability would indicate that regular visits to the doctor begin even before menstruation has stopped. Postmenopausal women who are in good health ought to have a checkup once a year.

HOW TO CHOOSE A DOCTOR

If you do not have a family doctor, finding one is not difficult. A call to the local medical society, listed in the telephone directory, will usually result in a number of names. While you will receive no recommendations, you can in this way obtain a list of doctors who practice in the community and who are in good standing in the local medical society.

You should specify that you wish a general practitioner, a family practitioner, or an internist. With the trend toward specialization in medicine, this may be a good place to clear up any confusion about these terms. A general practitioner is a doctor who usually has had little or no formal training after his one-year internship following graduation from medical school; he is not certified in a specialty of medicine and he usually treats all types of general medical problems.

A family practitioner also has a general practice, but current medical training now provides a residency and offers certification by the American Board of Family Practice in this specialty. A family practitioner is thus properly called a specialist, and the trend toward this type of training is growing in many areas of the country.

An internist or specialist in internal medicine has usually completed at least two years of a residency in medicine and may have additional training in one of the medical subspecialties like hematology or cardiology. Most but not all internists have passed a formal examination given by the American Board of Internal Medicine which certifies their competency in this specialty. If the letters F.A.C.P. follow your physician's name, he has passed the board examination and has also completed some additional scholarly work in the field to qualify as a Fellow of the American College of Physicians.

A cardiologist is a physician who has taken further training in heart disease and has passed the examination in the specific field of cardiology in addition to the one in medicine. If he has published some scholarly work in the field, he may also be a Fellow of the American College of Cardiology, entitled to use the initials F.A.C.C. after his name. (Some very competent cardiologists have not passed the formal board exams and may or may not be fellows of the American College of Cardiology.)

In general, it is wise for the individual not to shop around on his own for a superspecialist. For a general checkup and for most other adult problems either a general family practitioner or an internist is the best source of referral to the various specialties. In case of a serious problem, he can oversee the general management of the illness, pulling together the many skills that may be needed in time of trouble.

Judging the competence of a physician is not easy. In general, if a physician has been practicing in a community for more than a few years and if he has admitting privileges at a good local hospital, he is an adequate physician. Word of mouth is a powerful force and if you are new in a community or going to see a physician for the first time, you might ask around among your co-workers or neighbors. You can check a physician's training by asking the local medical society or by using the *Directory of American Medical Specialists,* published by the American Medical Association, which is available at most larger libraries.

Your relationship with your doctor is of prime importance, and I would urge you to select one with whom you are compatible. A good working relationship with a physician is composed of equal parts of respect, trust, and confidence along with a generous helping of affection. Hostility in the medical relationship is counter-productive, and if you do not get along with your doctor it is wise to find another.

WHAT A VISIT TO YOUR PHYSICIAN SHOULD TELL YOU

Your doctor will start the examination by taking a history; you will reply frankly and honestly. His knowledge of your background and your problem is crucial in his choice of treatment for you, so be sure that you withhold no information that may be of importance. A busy physician does not ask questions to pry and he cannot be expected to practice both medicine and omniscience. He will ask your age and occupation along with a pertinent family history. Has there been any premature coronary heart disease in your family? Other premature cardiovascular disease? Diabetes? Gout? If your parents are no longer living, what did they die of and at what age? The doctor will note any serious illnesses that you have had, along with a fairly detailed description of any hospitalization. In assessing your possible risk of heart trouble, he will be especially interested in the amount of physical work connected with your job and in your emotional reaction to your work—the stress it creates in your life.

In taking your history, the doctor will be interested in whether you smoke or drink and how much. He will want to know about your marital adjustment and any problems at home. He will ask about allergies and childhood diseases as well as any previous evidence of abnormalities in the digestive, genitourinary, or respiratory systems. The doctor will ask about your endocrine system in questions concerning your thyroid or the presence of diabetes. He will want to know about any blood disorders that you have had in the past as well as any impairment of the musculoskeletal or neurological systems.

With regard to your heart, the doctor will want to know of any evidence of high blood pressure, rheumatic fever, or heart murmurs. Any specific symptoms such as shortness of breath, chest pain, or chest discomfort should be noted and carefully described. Does it come on in the evening? With exertion or emotional or physical stress? With sexual excitement? Have you ever had chest pains at rest?

If you have been short of breath, the doctor will want to pin down the circumstances of its occurrence: Does it come on with exertion or at rest? How much activity is needed to produce the shortness of breath? When does it usually occur? Are you short of breath at night when you are lying flat in bed? During the day? After meals? If the breathing difficulty occurs at night your doctor will want to know whether it helps to lie on two or three pillows or whether it is necessary to get up and walk around a bit before the symptoms abate.

Your doctor will ask about palpitations, that strange sensation of a skipped heartbeat, or any "racing" that you have experienced. He will want to know whether you have ever felt a "flip-flopping" of the heart or the sensation that the heart is pumping very hard. He will also ask about any swelling of the feet or ankles.

THE PHYSICAL EXAMINATION

Following the history, the doctor will perform a complete physical examination. You should know that many important aspects of the physical are accomplished by the physician's keen awareness of the patient's appearance. As he observes you, the doctor is mentally noting how you walk, sit, and move; these signs are often valuable clues to various diseases. Your general state of health, whether robust or pallid, vibrant and communicative or withdrawn, energetic or fatigued are most immediately apparent. In some cases, the presence of certain cardiac conditions is suspected when the doctor notes that your skin or lips are blue-tinged or white and that your fingertips are pale in color.

The status of your nutrition and hydration will be seen from your general body build and the tightness of the skin. More detailed examination of the skin may reveal signs of cholesterol abnormalities in the form of yellow patches below the eyes or on the knees and elbows. The physician will observe your rate and type of breathing, often a valuable sign in detecting lung or heart disease. In these ways, the doctor can often tell as much from your outward physical appearance as he can from the more detailed part of the physical examination.

The physician will use his sense of touch, too, in an effort to pin down your exact physical condition. The laying on of hands frequently begins with the measurement of the pulse. In those fifteen to thirty seconds, the physician's hand on your wrist is counting the rate, noting whether your heartbeat is irregular, whether you have any extra beats, or whether your heart is too slow or too fast. He is also gauging the strength of the heart and judging whether the main valve is opening efficiently. All of these findings are clues that will be followed up on direct examination of the heart as well as with laboratory studies, x-rays, and electrocardiograms.

A most important part of the physical examination, especially with regard to the development of heart disease, is the measurement of the blood pressure. This determination is of special value because most patients with high blood pressure have no symptoms and are completely unaware of any abnormality. Hypertension, or high blood pressure, is an important risk factor and can easily and effectively be treated with little or no discomfort to the patient. If the physician finds that your blood pressure is elevated, he may wish to repeat the measurement later in the examination after you have become more relaxed or after you have sat quietly for a time. In many instances, if there is only a mild elevation he may ask you to return in a week or two for another blood pressure check before he starts a course of treatment designed to bring down the blood pressure.

During the remainder of the physical examination the physician will assess the present condition of your heart, lungs, abdomen, and other parts of the body. It is sometimes amazing to the patient that most of the information that is required for a physical examination can be obtained in less than ten minutes, especially if there are no abnormalities present. This is because the doctor uses a well-trained complex of judgments and responses that depend on his eyes, ears, and sense of touch and smell as well as the most accurate medical tool of all, his brain. A well-trained physician collects and filters the data presented by a complex human being in a rapid and efficient manner.

You, as the patient, can aid this process in several ways. If the doctor makes any comments in the course of the examination that you find frightening or difficult to understand, ask him to back up for a moment and explain them to you in detail. In this way you can alleviate a great deal of unnecessary anxiety and, in the process, insure that communication between you and your doctor remains open. This may also be a good place to test your selection of the physician, since it is essential that you understand each other fully.

From a good history and physical examination, the physician can assess your general health and can to a great extent determine the state of your heart. If no abnormalities of the heart are found —if it is of normal size, if the sounds are normal, and if there are no signs of heart failure and no history suggesting coronary artery disease or congestive failure—then there are other aspects of an examination that can supply some further clues as to the risk of heart attack. They include family history, individual history of cigarette smoking, blood pressure, presence or absence of lipid abnormalities as reflected in the levels of cholesterol in the blood, and obesity. These known coronary risk factors and what can be done about them are discussed in detail in subsequent chapters of this book.

LABORATORY STUDIES

In addition to the data obtained from the history and physical examination, laboratory tests are usually done on blood and urine samples to provide further information about the patient's current state of health and the efficiency of his heart function as well as his possible risk of developing heart disease.

Using these tests, the doctor rounds out his picture of the patient's general condition and determines the course of treatment, if any, as well as the appropriate program to prevent the possible development of heart disease. This underscores another good reason for seeing the physician for regular checkups: findings obtained when you are in good health serve as a base line against which any subsequent changes may be measured. This is especially important with regard to the chest x-ray and electrocardiogram.

In the usual medical practice a standard battery of blood tests is routinely ordered. You will probably be asked not to eat anything for at least eight hours prior to your appointment, in practice to have nothing but water after dinner the evening before. This is to insure that the blood sample drawn is not affected by your last meal. Even the carbohydrates in a cup of coffee with cream and a doughnut will throw off a number of the standard tests, and a martini prior to a late afternoon appointment will have even more conspicuous effects. Since not all the laboratory tests will be affected by what you may have recently eaten, it is important to let the doctor know if and when you may inadvertently have had a meal. He can take this into consideration when he analyzes the test results.

BLOOD COUNT

Your blood sample is first routinely analyzed for the amount of hemoglobin and the percentage of red blood cells it contains. The resulting *hematocrit* value indicates the oxygen-carrying capacity of the blood, important data in the diagnosis of a number of disease states. In terms of the heart, the anemia indicated by a low hematocrit or reduced hemoglobin content of the blood can cause minor coronary problems to become symptomatic. In some cases the symptoms of coronary artery disease can be relieved by the relatively simple process of treating the anemia to increase the amount of oxygen-carrying components in the bloodstream.

The finding of too many red cells can also be treated relatively easily. In order to keep the hematocrit or percentage of red blood cells within normal limits, the doctor can draw some blood periodically and in this way avoid the appearance of symptoms.

The number and condition of the white cells in the blood are also noted since they are of importance in a variety of systemic and blood diseases.

URINALYSIS

The doctor will usually ask for a sample of your urine for analysis. Patients sometimes worry that they may not be able to produce on cue, but I hasten to assure you that if you relax and take your time you can produce the small amount of urine needed for the routine studies. Physicians and nurses understand that a patient may have some occasional difficulty, and they will be happy to give the time you need.

Analysis of the urine provides a great deal of information about the functioning of the kidneys. The color of the urine, its specific gravity, the presence or absence of protein, and the number and types of cells are important clues to the physician who is seeking a complete picture of the patient's condition. Abnormal kidney function can result in hypertension and, if the blood pressure is found to be elevated, additional tests of kidney function may be ordered.

With regard to heart disease, a very important aspect of the urinalysis is the routine test for sugar. Sugar in the urine is a sign of diabetes and its presence suggests that measures for its control are necessary. Diabetes increases the risk of heart disease, and most physicians will want to treat it, either with diet or medication, as soon as it is diagnosed. Other risk factors are usually treated more vigorously if diabetes is present, and weight control becomes extremely important to the patient's good health.

BLOOD GLUCOSE LEVELS

In addition to the blood count, blood samples are usually analyzed for the presence or elevation of other substances, many of which can have an important bearing on the individual's risk of developing coronary heart disease. One of the most important is the blood glucose determination, which tests for sugar in the blood that may indicate the presence of diabetes even before sugar appears in the urine. If there is an abnormally high level in the blood, a glucose tolerance test may be done. Samples of blood are drawn at one-hour intervals after a measured glucose meal that is most often taken in the form of carbonated cola-flavored beverage. This sensitive test tells a great deal about the body's metabolism of sugar, and it may indicate the presence of covert or preclinical diabetes.

Diabetes is a serious metabolic disease that affects almost every part of the body. By using the standard blood tests your doctor can detect its presence long before enough sugar has built up in the bloodstream to spill over into the urine and he can institute effective measures for its control.

The detection of diabetes is extremely important in any examination because among its many harmful effects is the acceleration of the atherosclerotic process. For reasons still not completely known, diabetes affects the blood vessels in a way that results in the premature development of atherosclerosis. The coronary arteries are most often affected, and their narrowing sets the stage for a possible heart attack. Epidemiological studies have demonstrated that diabetes is frequently found among patients who develop coronary disease. Its early detection is important because measures for its control can be instituted as soon as it is confirmed.

Diabetes can often be controlled by diet alone; as a matter of fact some early forms in the obese can be completely suppressed by weight loss. In most of the remaining cases diet combined with glucose-lowering drugs or insulin will lead to prompt normalizing of the blood sugar. Since the tendency to diabetes is inherited and the disease does increase the individual risk of heart disease, your physician will consider abnormal glucose findings seriously. He will begin to control blood sugar levels with measures that are effective and comfortable; he may suggest some prophylactic steps to avoid the other complications of diabetes and he will certainly insist on weight loss if you are obese.

As is the case with so many other areas of medicine, modern research into the effects of controlling blood glucose levels has told us how much we still do not know. In this extremely complex condition, there is still considerable controversy over what effect controlling the blood sugar level by diet or insulin or both has on the development of atherosclerosis. In light of incontrovertible evidence that diabetics have a higher risk for heart attack than people without diabetes, most physicians institute treatment, especially weight loss and dietary control, as soon as the diagnosis is made.

The diet is usually restricted at once, lowering sugar intake to correct for the metabolic defect. Cholesterol and triglyceride levels are also attacked through diets that are low in saturated fats and carbohydrates since diabetics have a strong tendency toward abnormal lipid levels in the blood.

Your doctor will probably suggest strict control of the other risk factors as well. In the presence of a diabetic abnormality it is vital that blood pressure and cholesterol levels be kept within normal limits. Cigarette smoking should be halted at once. The coronary risk factors are known to be synergistic in their effects —each one both adds to and increases the importance of the other factors. A prudent individual, told that he has diabetes, either overt or preclinical, should respond with a lifelong determination to control all of the known coronary risk factors.

URIC ACID LEVELS AND GOUT

Uric acid is another of the chemical prognosticators of heart disease. Elevated uric acid levels in the blood are occasionally manifested by the development of gout, a painful inflammation of the joints caused by the presence of crystals of uric acid. Although the causal relationship of elevated uric acid levels to heart disease remains obscure, high uric acid levels are clearly associated with increased risk of heart attack. We are not sure that normalizing uric acid levels achieves the goal of decreasing the risk of heart disease, but there is little question that dietary or drug control of the condition is prudent.

If uric acid levels are found to be elevated in your blood, your physician may suggest a diet that restricts food high in purines, the chemical precursors of uric acid. These include legumes (beans, peas), organ meats, and small fish such as anchovies. Uric acid can also be lowered by drugs which either increase the amount excreted in the urine or block its formation in the body. An acute attack of gout is treated differently, the aim here being to cool the inflammation and control the pain.

Like the blood sugar, uric acid levels are found to be elevated in people who are constantly subjected to nervous strain, suggesting still another possible link in the chain that leads from stress to heart attacks. The biochemical picture is so complex that research may ultimately disclose that it is neither uric acid nor glucose itself that promotes the deposit of atherosclerotic plaque but rather some underlying metabolic defect that promotes the coincident development of all three.

BLOOD LIPIDS: CHOLESTEROL AND TRIGLYCERIDES

The blood tests directly associated with risk of heart attack are those that determine the level of *serum lipids* or fats found in the blood. In fact the control of the major blood lipids, *cholesterol* and *triglycerides,* is considered by many experts to be the most important part of any coronary prevention program. If premature heart disease is a part of your family background, or if you have cardiovascular symptoms of any kind, your physician may want to check and classify your lipid levels at a relatively early age. In certain cases it may be wise to examine the children, since certain more serious forms of elevated cholesterol are known to be familial.

The biochemistry of the lipids in the human bloodstream is complex. Fats are the storage form of fuel in the body. When we eat, the foods we ingest are broken down in the stomach and intestines into their simple components: carbohydrates (sugar and starches), proteins, and lipids or fats (including cholesterol, triglycerides, and others). These simple substances are absorbed through the intestinal wall into the bloodstream. Most of these components are delivered to the liver, a remarkable organ that acts both as a distribution center and a factory.

The components needed for fuel, mostly carbohydrates and fats, are released directly into the bloodstream and delivered to the cells of the body. The proteins or their components (called amino acids) are either delivered directly or used by the liver cells to manufacture other needed proteins. The fats and carbohydrates not needed for immediate use as fuel are not wasted but are either stored in the liver or changed so that they can be readily stored in other parts of the body. Most of the carbohydrate is changed to glycogen, a starchlike conglomeration of simple sugars that is stored in the liver for future use. The liver stores enough to supply the needs of the body for about twenty-four hours, in this way maintaining a constant level of sugar in the blood between meals. The carbohydrate that is left over and the fats that are not immediately used are changed into triglycerides, another form of fat, which are transported from the liver through the blood to the fat cells found just under the skin in almost all parts of the body. The fat cells take up this excess fuel and store it, usually in bulges, until it is needed. If much more fat is taken in than can be used, the stores accumulate and obesity develops.

Now aside from accounting for the buildup of fat, the transport of these triglycerides from the liver to the fat cells for storage (and back to the liver for reconversion to more useful fuels when needed) forms an important part of the body's economy. The carrier substance that effects these transfers is called a *lipoprotein* and it is manufactured in the liver. Cholesterol, which in small amounts is also necessary in the production of certain hormones and of the bile salts, forms a major part of this carrier lipoprotein and as such is of basic importance. Most of the cholesterol in the blood is in the form of this carrier lipoprotein.

Abnormally high levels of cholesterol in the blood are due to overproduction or decreased breakdown of these lipoproteins. An increased blood triglyceride level is due either to an excess being picked up from the liver or to an inadequate release of the triglyceride from the carrier protein. Although the body can manufacture cholesterol if it is needed, most of the cholesterol in the blood originates from the animal fats present in the food we eat. This is especially true in people who have a tendency toward high cholesterol levels; the amount of dietary cholesterol needed for health is not entirely known but it is felt to be virtually nil.

TYPES OF ELEVATED BLOOD LIPID LEVELS

Abnormally high cholesterol and triglyceride levels have been correlated strongly with the occurrence of coronary artery disease. If these lipids are found to be elevated in the standard blood test, your doctor may decide to learn more about your particular abnormality by ordering a *lipoprotein electrophoresis*. This blood test identifies the specific type of abnormality, and data obtained from these very detailed studies allow the doctor to make certain inferences about the relation of the lipid abnormality to coronary disease.

Using the patterns provided by electrophoresis, the physician can then "type" the specific lipid abnormality. (The biochemical composition of the various types of abnormalities and the specific treatment of each is given in Chapter 6, "Cholesterol and Triglycerides.")

Type II is characterized by high levels of cholesterol; Type IV by high triglyceride levels; Type III is a rare type with high levels of both cholesterol and triglyceride; and CHL-combined hyperlipidemia is a more common elevation of both. Knowing the specific type of hyperlipidemia, the doctor can tailor a program that is known to be effective in the specific control needed. Although all of these lipid abnormalities are probably due to defects in the lipid transport process, most can be successfully treated with dietary manipulation and weight loss, if obesity is present.

Recently it has been demonstrated that the amount of one of the normal lipoproteins in the blood is inversely related to the individuals' risk of developing coronary artery disease. The substance, high density lipoprotein (HDL), tends to be high in patients with no coronary disease and low in those with coronary disease. The level of HDL is measured by separating out the part of the blood in which the HDL is found and then measuring the cholesterol in that fraction. (The cholesterol content of HDL is relatively constant.) This measurement is reported as the HDL cholesterol, but comprises only a small amount of the total cholesterol in the blood. This term is unfortunate because it has generated the belief that there is "good" and "bad" cholesterol. If the total blood cholesterol level is abnormally elevated it is virtually always due to cholesterol in the lipoproteins associated with coronary disease and rarely due to elevated HDL levels.

In most cases any detrimental lipid elevation that is seen will be relatively slight, and from his knowledge of you and your family your doctor may conclude that it can be treated with only a moderate degree of dietary restriction. He will also want to check to determine that the blood lipid elevation is not due to the presence of alcohol or some other drug, the effects of diabetes, or the use of hormones such as estrogen.

By supplying a diet tailored to your particular lipid problem, your doctor will have taken only the first step. He will point out that only you can determine what goes into your mouth; he will probably suggest that stress is known to elevate cholesterol levels and in certain selected cases he may prescribe a cholesterol-lowering drug. But you will note that all of these measures leave the ball firmly in your court. In the last analysis, it is only you who can effect any change in the level of fats in your bloodstream.

Knowing that high cholesterol is associated with disease and that it has been shown in several studies that lowered levels bring down the expected rate of heart attack; knowing that cholesterol-lowering measures have been endorsed by all of the leading health associations in the United States, including the American Heart Association and the American Medical Association; and knowing that most American doctors try at least to reduce dietary cholesterol in their own families, the prudent person will heed the signal flashed by an abnormal lipid finding and will embark on the simple measures suggested by his physician. More detailed information on cholesterol and its control is given in Chapter 6.

LIVER FUNCTION TESTS

The small sample of blood that you surrender to the technician on entering the doctor's office may also be tested for the presence of certain enzymes. In general these relate to the function of the liver and your doctor may wish to have the results of these studies as part of your base-line record.

The enzyme tests, which in the normal patient are related to liver function, are done routinely in case of a definite or suspected heart attack because they will indicate the presence and extent of damage in the cells of the heart. Knowing the normal levels obtained at the time of an earlier office visit may thus prove valuable should your physician wish to make a comparison.

BLOOD-UREA-NITROGEN (BUN)

Another routinely done test is the blood-urea-nitrogen determination or BUN. The results of this test relate generally to kidney function and may also be related to the presence of hypertension. Again as part of the record it helps your physician to evaluate any changes that may appear at a later date.

CHEST X-RAY

A chest x-ray should be included in a routine check-up. In the absence of symptoms this is usually done no more than once a year. A painless and rapidly completed procedure, the chest x-ray is useful in revealing abnormalities in the lungs such as tuberculosis, pneumonia, or the start of lung cancer.

In terms of possible heart disease the chest x-ray is useful in the diagnosis and documentation of certain conditions. Any enlargement of the heart can be seen and, if congestive heart failure is suspected, the findings of the chest x-ray will be of great value. Again, if there are symptoms of heart disease or if a cardiac abnormality is suspected on the basis of the routine chest x-ray, a more detailed cardiac series may be done to pinpoint the exact problem.

Occasionally if an abnormality appears in the chest x-ray or if a heart murmur is heard, fluoroscopy of the heart is done. The patient stands behind a screen and the doctor uses x-ray equipment to watch movement of the heart. Fluoroscopy provides additional information about the valves and allows the doctor to view the contraction sequence of the beating heart.

THE ELECTROCARDIOGRAM

Modern electrocardiography has to be considered one of the most important diagnostic tools in cardiology today. Painless, accurate, and easily done, the electrocardiogram or ECG tracing provides information about the function and integrity of the heart by sensing the polarization and depolarization across the membranes of the heart cells and by measuring the differences in voltage among the various parts of the body where the leads are placed. The electric charge is recorded by a sensitive galvanometer that is similar in principle to those commonly used in radio repair shops and, because the charge is slight, electronic equipment is used to amplify and record the signal on paper tape specially marked to note the timing of the sequence.

The line the ECG traces at a known speed on graph paper has little meaning except when it is interpreted by a trained physician and considered together with the other findings that constitute your record. Its value lies in the fact that, before any part of the heart contracts, there are electrical changes in each of the cells of the heart. By recording these changes, the ECG yields information of various types.

First, the rhythm of the heart and its rate can be determined by the placement of the peaks and valleys on the tracing. Abnormally fast or slow rhythms can be picked up at once, as can evidence of skipped beats, dropped beats, or irregular rhythms. The physician can also make inferences about the origin of rhythm disturbances from the evidence seen on the ECG.

The electrocardiogram also traces the sequence of the contraction of the heart. In the normal pattern, the left and right atria contract simultaneously just before the simultaneous contraction of the right and left ventricles. If there is an abnormal delay between the contraction of the atria and the ventricles or between the contraction of the two ventricles, this too appears on the ECG. Any enlargement of the walls of the four chambers of the heart can be detected on the ECG, as can any damage that may have been caused in the past by a "silent" heart attack which may have caused only minimal symptoms. If ischemia is present— that is, if the oxygen supply to any part of the heart is inadequate —it too can be diagnosed from a routine electrocardiogram.

Since it provides all of this information, it is easy to see why an electrocardiogram taken during good health can serve as a base line to which an ECG taken during an episode of any kind can be compared. By looking at both tracings, the doctor can frequently determine the nature of any problem that may have developed between the two electrocardiograms.

What your doctor *cannot* tell from a normal electrocardiogram is whether you are going to have a heart attack in the near future. Invaluable for determining the present condition or past history of the heart, the ECG has only limited value as a prognosticator. For this reason everyone knows of someone who died soon after being pronounced sound by his doctor; unfortunately, the ECG can only hint at what will occur in the future.

On rare occasions, the ECG appears to be normal in the presence of fairly widespread coronary artery disease; in these cases, the clogging of the arteries, though severe, for some reason does not appear to affect the routine ECG. This occurs primarily because the ECG can only demonstrate either damaged heart muscle or ischemia that is occurring at the time that the test is performed. If there has been no heart muscle damage and the patient is not having ischemia the record may be normal. There are also other reasons for a normal ECG in the presence of severe coronary disease. To determine the exact cause of certain symptoms, therefore, specialized electrocardiography is sometimes done in the doctor's office or in the heart station of a modern hospital.

STRESS TESTING

In some instances the doctor will want to know how your electrocardiogram is affected by a measured amount of stress placed on the heart. The classical method is the Master's Two-Step Test, during which the patient exercises by walking up and down a two-step apparatus a certain number of times.

Either the treadmill test, where the patient walks on a moving belt at increasingly rapid speeds and increasing grades, or the bicycle ergometer test, where the patient pedals a specially equipped exercise bicycle for a fixed period or until the heart rate reaches a predetermined level, is more commonly used today.

The doctor monitors the patient carefully during the test, observing the ECG taken during the testing as well as the ECG done several minutes after the stress has ended. Physical exercise increases the demand on the heart, requiring it to work harder and to use more oxygen. If there is not sufficient blood flow or if the coronary arteries are too narrowed by atherosclerosis to allow this increase in supply, even if the blood flow is adequate during rest, certain telltale changes will appear on the ECG. By observing the patient's symptoms and blood pressure changes and by noting carefully the pattern of ECG changes and the amount of stress required to produce them, the doctor can gain important insight into the adequacy of the patient's coronary blood flow.

Although accurate in most instances, false positive tests (positive results in patients with normal coronaries) and false negative tests may occur. False positive tests are especially common in women and are not uncommon in men who have no symptoms. Depending on the clinical findings and how strongly positive the stress test is, your physician may suggest further more sophisticated testing such as coronary arteriography.

LONG-TERM ELECTROCARDIOGRAPHIC MONITORING (HOLTER MONITORING)

There is another electrocardiographic technique used to solve the mystery of symptoms in people whose office or resting ECG appears to be normal. This method of long-term continuous electrocardiography requires that the patient wear a small portable device that records the ECG on tape during six to twenty-four hours of normal activity. The equipment for long-term continuous electrocardiography is manufactured by several different firms but the original system was described by Dr. Norman Holter in 1957.

In current office practice, a patient complaining of dizziness, fainting, palpitations, or chest pain is first evaluated carefully by the standard resting electrocardiogram, possibly on several occasions. If repeated office ECGs fail to give enough information to make a diagnosis, the patient can be fitted with a portable device.

The equipment weighs about one pound, is entirely external, and can be worn comfortably under clothing. The tapes vary in size, recording from six to twenty-four hours of the heart's electrical activity. It should be noted that twelve hours of continuous recording yields *seventy thousand* cardiac cycles, as compared to the fifty or sixty recorded by the standard office ECG. Portable monitoring equipment allows the collection of data on the heart's function during the patient's usual activities, and it is invaluable in the diagnosis of conditions that may appear only during specific activities—for example, during commuting or while at work.

The tapes are run at high speed through advanced equipment using visual scanners and computers to plot any abnormalities occurring during the recorded period. Evaluated by the physician, who correlates them with his other findings, these data facilitate the proper diagnosis of what may be an extremely important but transient disturbance. For patients with symptoms such as chest pain or shortness of breath but who have normal resting electrocardiograms, and in those for whom exercise testing provides no further clues, six- to twenty-four-hour ambulatory monitoring is an especially valuable diagnostic tool.

Sometimes symptoms like palpitations, dizziness, or fainting spells are caused by short episodes of extremely slow heart rates or inordinately fast heart rates that may not appear on a routine ECG when done in the physician's office. When continuous ECG recording reveals episodes of lowered heart rates, the doctor may elect to insert a permanent pacemaker to control and modulate the heart rate. If rapid abnormal rhythms are noted, the proper drug therapy can be instituted.

Long-term ECG (LCG) monitoring also allows the physician to assess the effect of drugs given to control arrhythmias (PVCs or premature ventricular contractions), adjusting the dosage according to the heart's responses over a six- to twenty-four-hour period.

In patients with known coronary heart disease or in those who have already suffered a myocardial infarction, LCG provides a great deal of information on the course of the disease. Some physicians now feel that all heart attack victims should be monitored for at least twelve hours just before their discharge from the hospital. In the hospital setting the physician may use a telemetry system allowing the patient to wear a portable device that changes the ECG to radio waves that are transmitted to a receiver in the coronary care unit and monitored on line. The ECG produced during this period of relative activity can supply important clues as to the medical management of the patient as well as to his probable risk of difficulty in the months following the acute event.

In the postmyocardial infarction patient, LCG is used to evaluate the response to work activity, especially if there is some difficulty on the job. By recording the heart's responses during a normal day that includes work, play, and relaxation, the LCG gives important guidelines to what does and what does not produce electrocardiographic changes. Long-term ECG monitoring may also prove useful in evaluating people with a strong family history of coronary heart disease or those who may be at high risk for one of the other coronary risk factors.

A newly developed form of long-term monitor records sample ECGs once or twice an hour. An abnormal rhythm will trigger the device, and some units also allow the patient to activate the recorder as soon as symptoms appear. Monitoring equipment of this kind, worn over a long period of time, enables the doctor to see what the electrocardiogram looks like when the patient is having his difficulties.

VECTORCARDIOGRAM

If more information on the electrical activity of the heart is needed for diagnosis or treatment, the doctor may order a sophisticated study called the *vector cardiogram*. Like the routine ECG, the vector cardiogram measures the electrical changes associated with the heart's contraction, but it possesses the additional ability of giving a two-dimensional picture. While the routine electrocardiogram measures the electrical forces in one direction, the vector cardiogram measures the forces in two perpendicular directions at the same time, in this way giving considerably more information than a standard ECG. The vector cardiogram is displayed on an oscilloscope, a viewing device much like a television screen, which shows detailed pictures of the electrical forces in three planes of the heart—horizontal, sagittal, and frontal.

Like the routine electrocardiogram, the vector cardiogram is a completely safe and painless procedure. It requires only that the patient remain still for about ten minutes while a number of electrodes and mysterious looking wires are placed across his chest, down his back, on his limbs, and on his forehead. The total effect is one of science fiction, but I can assure you that the procedure is very valuable in pinpointing the significance of certain abnormalities.

PHONOCARDIOGRAM

If the physician hears abnormal heart sounds or heart murmurs during the physical examination, he may order a phonocardiogram.

The phonocardiogram is a sophisticated electronic device that is used to check further into any unusual heart sounds. Murmurs, gallops, or extra sounds are all important sometimes in determining whether disease or impairment may be present. The phonocardiogram amplifies and records the heart sounds and produces a graphic representation that is useful in diagnosing anything unusual that may have been heard through the stethoscope.

The heart sounds are picked up by a small microphone placed on the chest and the sounds are converted electronically into a visual display and recorded on a running paper strip. The doctor can then correlate the presence of the sound with the contraction of the heart as it appears on the electrocardiogram, along with other wave forms that are recorded at the same time. These include the pulse in one of the two main arteries in the neck, the carotid artery, the pulse in the large vein in the neck, and the apex cardiogram, the pulse that is felt directly over the heart. The configuration of these pulses is also valuable in determining the integrity of the heart valves and the strength and function of the heart muscle.

ECHOCARDIOGRAM

The technology needed to develop the echocardiogram came to us from the unlikely source of submarine warfare. Like the sonar used by sub-chasers to detect the presence of submarines in the area, the echocardiogram senses and records reflected sound waves. The transducer that the doctor holds in his hand both emits a very high-pitched inaudible sound and senses the sounds reflected from the heart. Extremely advanced electronic equipment converts the sound and displays it on an oscilloscopic screen that allows the doctor to visualize the fine structures of the heart and their movement.

The echocardiogram can detect very small changes in density; movements of the heart muscle, the valve leaflets, and the pericardium can be recorded and studied using equipment that is entirely external, safe, and painless. Echocardiography is a relatively new development in cardiology and all of its uses have not yet been fully defined. So far the echocardiogram has proved of great value in the exact diagnosis of abnormal fluid around the heart in the pericardium, in delineating valve abnormalities, and in diagnosing certain congenital abnormalities. The echocardiogram may prove to be most useful in pointing out areas where the poor contraction pattern of the heart suggests some difficulty with coronary blood flow.

All of these tests are safe, painless, and extremely valuable. Your physician may request them in order to pin down a diagnosis and to judge the effectiveness of treatment. Advanced and sophisticated, these modern electronic techniques should produce no anxiety in the patient. More often than not, these noninvasive tests —done from outside the body—yield important information that formerly could be obtained only with more hazardous surgical measures, if at all.

ESTIMATING YOUR RISK OF HEART ATTACK

When your physician has completed your work-up and evaluated the results of your laboratory studies, he will probably want to discuss his findings with you. At this time he will point out any abnormalities that he has found and he will suggest the measures that he wants you to follow for their correction or treatment. If you are obese he will probably suggest weight loss; if you are a smoker he almost certainly will ask you to stop or cut down significantly. If your examination indicates that you are diabetic or hypertensive the physician will suggest a specific regimen that you must follow —diet, certain drugs, or a way of life that will constitute therapy for the control of these factors. The same thing is true if elevated cholesterol or uric acid levels are found. If your physician does not mention aspects of risk of heart disease, or if there is anything that you do not understand, be certain to ask him about them. It is necessary that the patient understand fully the findings of his examination, and your physician will expect you to ask for clarification so that you can follow his instructions with insight and good judgment.

The American Heart Association has performed a valuable service in providing the physician with convenient tables that he can use in daily practice to estimate a patient's risk of heart disease. Contained in the AHA's publication, *The Coronary Risk Handbook,* these tables were derived from the data generated by the Framingham study and are considered valid for most of the population of the United States. Although the material contained in these tables reflects the experience of a group rather than of an individual, your physician can derive a figure from them that gives a rough estimate of your probability of developing coronary heart disease within a six-year period.

The Coronary Risk Handbook is available to your physician through the American Heart Association. Organized by sex and age group, the tables yield a number that reflects the probability of developing coronary heart disease within six years in chances per hundred.

By considering the patient's age, sex, smoking history, electrocardiogram, and disposition to glucose intolerance (evidence of diabetes), the physician obtains a figure that can be considered a rough guide to individual risk. Other factors such as overweight, lack of physical activity, stress, and elevation of blood lipids other than cholesterol would increase the risk of heart attack in ways not easily quantified.

FINAL RISK FACTOR (FRF) FOR ONE HYPOTHETICAL PATIENT

The South Central Pennsylvania affiliate of the American Heart Association has developed work sheets that the physician may also use as a convenient record of the patient's risk of coronary heart disease. Reproduced with their permission is a data form and work sheet (Figure 4-1) that we have completed for a hypothetical patient.

The patient is a thirty-nine-year-old male whose weight of 190 pounds makes him more than 20 percent above his ideal weight. He has a sedentary job but walks part way to work each day. He has no known diseases, although he reports that his father died as a result of a stroke. Our hypothetical patient does not smoke; his cholesterol is 265 mg %; his blood sugar is 98 mg %; his ECG is normal and his blood pressure is one hundred thirty over eighty. As calculated on the work sheet on page 71, this patient's final risk factor (FRF) is 12.75. He would be considered at average risk for coronary heart disease and would be followed rather routinely.

Note, however, what happens if our hypothetical patient begins to smoke heavily, a pack or more each day. As recorded on the work sheet on page 71, his blood pressure might go up, with smoking, to 145/90. Cholesterol levels might also rise to 285 mg %. With just these two changes, both likely in heavy smokers, this

Name and Address

| Ht. | Wt. | Age | Sex |

DATA FORM AND WORK SHEET

							Minor / Major Factor
Sex-Age	Female under 45 **0.8**	Female 45 **1.25**	Male under 40 **1**	Female 45 and above **1.5**	Female over 45 **1.5**	Male over 55 **1.5**	Minor Factor
Percent of Standard Wt.	**High**	91-120 **1**	1 Mo? **1.25**	Completely Sedentary			Minor Factor
Physical Exercise				Completely Sedentary			Minor Factor
Known Disease (Record only the Highest one)	None **1**	Diabetes **1.5**	Diabetes **1.5**	High Blood Pressure **2**	Angina **2** Heart Attack **2**	Chest Pain followed by **1.5**	Minor Factor
Family History of Disease Encircle parent, sister, brother (Record only highest one)	None **1**	Diabetes **1.5**	High Blood Pressure **2**	High Blood Pressure **2**	Angina Heart Attack or Failure 50 or over	Angina, Heart Attack or Failure Under 50 (Parent or Sib)	Minor Factor
Smoking	Non-Smoker **1**	Cigars, Pipe or Cigarettes **1.5**	Cigarettes 20-30 Per Day	Cigarettes 40 or more per day			Major Factor
Cholesterol	199 mg % or less **1**	200-249 mg % **1.5**	250-280 mg % **2**	281 mg % or greater	Value from LAB		Major Factor
Glucose	109 mg % or less **1**	110-149 mg % (borderline) **1.5**	150-169 mg % (Diabetic) **2.5**	170 mg % or greater	Value from LAB		Major Factor
EKG	Normal or Slightly Suspicious **1**	Suspicious **2**	Definitely Abnormal **3**	Write in 2 or 3 Abnormality			Major Factor
Blood Pressure	Less than 140/95 **1**	140/96 to 160/105 **1.5**	160/101 to 220/110	Greater than 220/110	Measured B. P.	Allow Leeway of 20 mm Systolic and Adhere to Absolute Diastolic	Major Factor
							Final Risk Factor

GUIDE FOR FRF:

9.8 - 11.0	Below Average
11.1 - 14.0	Average
14.1 - 16.0	Above Average
16.1 - and above	High
	Report to Doctor and patient to be made in these terms.	Check one above

Note:
Add factors to obtain FRF.
If necessary, modify FRF according to your judgement

Refer to Family Doctor if:
FRF is above average or higher — or 2 or more Major Risk Factors are rated 2 or higher

(Encircle)
REFERRED   YES   NO

South Central Pennsylvania Heart Association
2915 Wayne Street, Harrisburg, Pa. 17111

71

patient's risk of coronary heart disease would be considerably higher and he might require specific help in controlling the risk factors of cigarette smoking, hypertension, and high cholesterol.

RISKO

The activities of the American Heart Association are wide ranging and imaginative, and the efforts of this outstanding organization should be supported by everyone. Their concern with the prevention of heart disease has led them to develop and supply material that should be read by everyone and I urge each reader to contact his local heart association for a list of booklets.

The Michigan affiliate of the American Heart Association has developed the available coronary risk factor material into a game called RISKO (Figure 4–3) that can be used by the individual to calculate his probable risk of heart atttack. With their permission I have reproduced RISKO.

If your score is 35 or above, you should make an appointment to see your physician and discuss with him possible measures to modify the specific factors that increase your risk of coronary heart disease.

RISKO and all other tabular material of this kind can provide only a rough estimate of probable risk, but the goal of prevention is so important and the role of the risk factors so vital that everyone can benefit from a yearly game of RISKO.

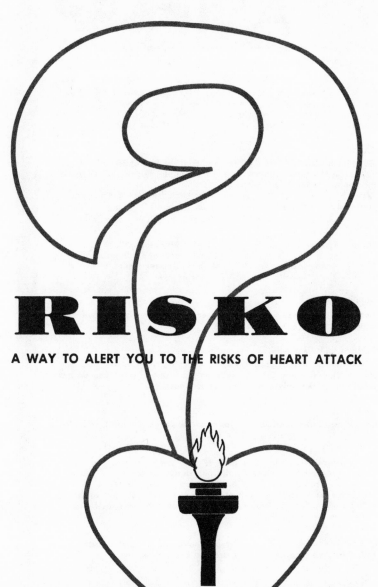

RISKO

A WAY TO ALERT YOU TO THE RISKS OF HEART ATTACK

DON'T PLAY GAMES WITH YOUR HEART. SEE YOUR DOCTOR
REGULARLY AND LET HIM HELP YOU REDUCE
YOUR RISK OF HEART ATTACK

73

RISKO

The purpose of this game is to give you an estimate of your chances of suffering heart attack.

The game is played by making squares which — from left to right — represent an increase in your RISK FACTORS. These are medical conditions and habits associated with an increased danger of heart attack. *Not all risk factors are measurable enough to be included in this game; see back of sheet for other RISK FACTORS.*

RULES:

Study each RISK FACTOR AND its row. Find the box applicable to you and circle the large number in it. For example, if you are 37, circle the number in the box labeled 31-40.
After checking out all the rows, add the circled numbers. This total — your score — is an estimate of your risk.

IF YOU SCORE:

6-11 — Risk well below
  average
12-17 — Risk below average
18-24 — Risk generally average

25-31 — Risk moderate
32-40 — Risk at a dangerous level
41-62 — Danger urgent. See your
  doctor now.

HEREDITY:

Count parents, grand-parents, brothers, and sisters who have had heart attack and/or stroke.

TOBACCO SMOKING:

If you inhale deeply and smoke a cigarette way down, add one to your classification. Do NOT subtract because you think you do not inhale or smoke only a half inch on a cigarette.

EXERCISE:

Lower your score one point if you exercise regularly and frequently.

CHOLESTEROL OR SATURATED FAT INTAKE LEVEL:

A cholesterol blood level is best. If you can't get one from your doctor, then estimate honestly the percentage of solid fats you eat. These are usually of animal origin — lard, cream, butter, and beef and lamb fat. If you eat much of this, your cholesterol level probably will be high. The U.S. average, 40%, is too high for good health.

BLOOD PRESSURE:

If you have no recent reading but have passed an insurance or industrial examination chances are you are 140 or less.

SEX:

This line takes into account the fact that men have from 6 to 10 times more heart attacks than women of child bearing age.

	1	2	3	4	6	8
AGE	**1** 10 to 20	**2** 21 to 30	**3** 31 to 40	**4** 41 to 50	**6** 51 to 60	**8** 61 to 70 and over
HEREDITY	**1** No known history of heart disease	**2** 1 relative with cardiovascular disease Over 60	**3** 2 relatives with cardiovascular disease Over 60	**4** 1 relative with cardiovascular disease Under 60	**6** 2 relatives with cardiovascular disease Under 60	**8** 3 relatives with cardiovascular disease Under 60
WEIGHT	**0** More than 5 lbs. below standard weight	**1** −5 to +5 lbs. standard weight	**2** 6-20 lbs. over weight	**3** 21-35 lbs. over weight	**5** 36-50 lbs. over weight	**7** 51-65 lbs. over weight
TOBACCO SMOKING	**0** Non-user	**1** Cigar and/or pipe	**2** 10 cigarettes or less a day	**4** 20 cigarettes a day	**6** 30 cigarettes a day	**10** 40 cigarettes a day or more
EXERCISE	**1** Intensive occupational and recreational exertion	**2** Moderate occupational and recreational exertion	**3** Sedentary work and intense recreational exertion	**5** Sedentary occupational and moderate recreational exertion	**6** Sedentary work and light recreational exertion	**8** Complete lack of all exercise
CHOLES-TEROL OR FAT % IN DIET	**1** Cholesterol below 180 mg.% Diet contains no animal or solid fats	**2** Cholesterol 181-205 mg.% Diet contains 10% animal or solid fats	**3** Cholesterol 206-230 mg.% Diet contains 20% animal or solid fats	**4** Cholesterol 231-255 mg.% Diet contains 30% animal or solid fats	**5** Cholesterol 256-280 mg.% Diet contains 40% animal or solid fats	**6** Cholesterol 281-300 mg.% Diet contains 50% animal or solid fats
BLOOD PRESSURE	**1** 100 upper reading	**2** 120 upper reading	**3** 140 upper reading	**4** 160 upper reading	**6** 180 upper reading	**8** 200 or over upper reading
SEX	**1** Female under 40	**2** Female 40-50	**3** Female over 50	**5** Male	**6** Stocky male	**7** Bald stocky male

Affiliate: American Heart Association
Member: Michigan United Fund
Torch Drive Agency

Michigan Heart Association

P.O. BOX L-V 160
16310 WEST TWELVE MILE ROAD
SOUTHFIELD, MICHIGAN 48076
313-557-9500

Because of the difficulty in measuring them, these RISK FACTORS are not included in "RISKO":

Diabetes, particularly when present for many years.

Your Character or Personality, and the Stress under which you live.

Vital Capacity — determined by measuring the amount of air you can take into your lungs in proportion to the size of your lungs. The less air you can breathe, the higher your risk.

Electrocardiogram — if certain abnormalities are present in the record of the electrical currents generated by your heart you have a higher risk.

Gout — is caused by a higher than normal amount of uric acid in the blood. Patients have an increased risk.

IF YOU HAVE A NUMBER OF RISK FACTORS, FOR THE SAKE OF YOUR HEALTH, ASK YOUR DOCTOR TO CHECK YOUR MEDICAL CONDITIONS AND QUIT YOUR RISK FACTOR HABITS.

NOTE: *The fact that various habits or conditions may be rated similarly in this test does not mean these are of equal risk. The reaction of individual human beings to Risk Factors — as to many other things — is so varied it is impossible to draw valid conclusions for any individual.*

This scale has been developed only to highlight what the Risk Factors are and what can be done about them. It is not designed to be a medical diagnosis.

Chapter 5

Hypertension: The Urgent Need to Control High Blood Pressure

Hypertension—high blood pressure—is the most tantalizingly promising of all the risk factors that predispose an individual to coronary artery disease and heart attacks. It is at once the most prevalent risk factor, the one that is most easily detected and most comfortably treated, and the one in which the rewards of treatment toward the goal of preventing heart attacks have been most promising.

Yet, because these facts are not widely known or acted upon, hypertension is the most frustrating of the risk factors. Although the American Heart Association has estimated that more than 23 million people in the United States have high blood pressure, most of them are not aware of it; among those who know they have hypertension, the overwhelming majority do not seek or continue effective treatment.

It is even more frustrating to consider the enormous potential benefits of adequate treatment in light of the twenty-five thousand deaths attributed each year directly to hypertension and the 1.5 million heart attacks and strokes occurring each year that may be indirectly due to long-standing high blood pressure. Almost two-thirds of those who suffer heart attacks are found to have high blood pressure, usually untreated. And, among people having strokes, a whopping three-fourths have high blood pressure.

The waste of individual lives and well-being is all the more unconscionable when we consider that the treatment of hypertension is, in most cases, easy and comfortable, with few side effects and very little inconvenience to the patient.

Most studies show that treatable high blood pressure is remarkably widespread. Even seasoned health professionals have recently been amazed to learn that at least 10 percent of any given population will on examination prove to have hypertension. In some areas the rate is much higher because blacks tend to have more widespread elevations in blood pressure than whites. A citywide screening in New Orleans in mid-1973 yielded a record discovery rate of more than 30 percent; that is, approximately one person out of every three who was examined proved to have hypertension.

The rate of treatment is lower still. When the problem was studied in a large population in Chicago, half of those found to be hypertensive had no idea that they had a condition that warranted immediate medical treatment. Less than half of those who knew of their condition were being treated, and only about half of those were receiving what most doctors would define as adequate therapy. Some rapid arithmetic based on these figures would indicate that only about one-eighth of any hypertensive population can be said to have its high blood pressure levels under adequate medical control.

The Treatment of Hypertension

Although the picture is now changing rapidly, there was a time when doctors disagreed at exactly what point high blood pressure should be treated. Until recent years, moreover, there were only a limited number of drugs available for treatment. More recent studies and newly developed methods of treatment have almost definitely concluded that *all* elevated blood pressure should be treated. Study after study has demonstrated with certainty that people with untreated hypertension suffer serious damage to the heart, brain, and kidneys at a much higher rate than do those whose blood pressure is controlled. Current medical techniques are safe, effective, and comfortable; with today's knowledge there is no reason whatever to delay or discontinue treatment.

The major reason why hypertension is so poorly controlled

in this country relates to the patient in two ways. First, hypertension is usually asymptomatic. Although headaches, frequent nosebleeds, dizziness, tinnitus, or ringing in the ears, and feelings of unsteadiness may indicate the presence of hypertension, none of these symptoms need occur even in the presence of significantly elevated blood pressure levels.

Symptoms of hypertension are also nonspecific. A recent study compared a group of people with hypertension to a matched group whose blood pressure levels were within the normal range. To no one's surprise, the symptoms of headache and dizziness were found to be as common in the normal group as they were among the hypertensives. The rarity of specific complaints underlines the need for regular physical checkups and for communitywide screening to identify the vast numbers of people who simply do not know that they have hypertension.

Another reason for the lack of adequate treatment has been some misunderstanding on the part of the patient, much of it derived from the fact that few people know that hypertension must be considered a lifelong condition. Once detected, high blood pressure is usually easily controlled, but it must be treated with varying dosages in most cases for the remainder of the patient's life. In most cases, however, treatment can be medically conservative and quite comfortable. And since hypertension has been found in some large epidemiologic studies to be the risk factor with the highest correlation for heart disease, and since it also predisposes the patient to other life-threatening conditions such as stroke and severe kidney disease, clearly every medical effort toward its control must be made.

DIAGNOSIS OF HYPERTENSION

When the doctor wraps the familiar cuff of the ubiquitous blood pressure apparatus around your upper arm, he is performing a most useful diagnostic test. As he pumps air into this instrument, the cuff inflates and the pressure it measures appears as a number on a gauge or as an elevation of a column of mercury. This occurs because the large artery in the arm is compressed as the cuff inflates and blood flow is cut off. The doctor listens with his stethoscope to the artery below the point of compression. As he slowly releases the pressure in the cuff he can hear exactly when the blood begins to flow again through the artery. This is the maximum pressure produced by the heart during its working or *systole* phase and is known as the *systolic pressure*. It is expressed in millimeters as the level of a column of mercury.

To determine the *diastolic pressure,* the level of blood pressure in the arterial system between heart contractions, the doctor listens until the sound of the distinct heartbeat disappears and the blood courses freely through the artery. These numbers are expressed as systolic over diastolic, or about 130/80 in the normal situation.

During systole the heart is in its working or contraction phase as the left ventricle pumps blood out through the aortic valve and into the arteries, producing the systolic pressure. When the valve closes the pressure in the aorta or the systemic circulation drops below the pressure required for ejection and the heart is in its resting or *diastole* phase. The pressure during diastole remains at a fairly high level of 60 to 90 millimeters of mercury because it would waste a great deal of energy to start the system up again if the pressure were allowed to drop to zero. In a wisdom of economy the body utilizes the elasticity always present in the walls of the aorta and the arteries to maintain this reduced pressure between contractions. Stretched during systole (heart contraction), this elasticity allows the blood to flow at reduced pressure during diastole or relaxation of the heart. The energy of the stretch of the arteries and the aorta is transmitted to the blood and causes continued forward flow, producing both the systolic and diastolic pressures.

As in any closed fluid system, the blood pressure depends on the rate of flow (the amount of blood being pumped out of the heart) and on the size of the vascular bed that the blood is being pumped into. The system can be compared to your garden hose: water pressure in the hose can be stepped up by increasing the amount of water coming from the faucet or by narrowing the gauge of the hose. Pressure can be decreased if the amount of water coming from the faucet is reduced or if the gauge of the hose widened. In just the same way, in the cardiovascular system the blood pressure will rise if flow is increased or if the blood vessels that receive the blood are constricted. If the blood flow decreases or the vessels open up and dilate, the blood pressure will go down.

Blood pressure in humans depends on two factors: the cardiac output, defined as the amount of blood pumped by the heart through the vascular system per minute, and on the amount of constriction or resistance present in the peripheral arteries. The cardiac output is determined by the strength of contraction of the heart, its rate, and, most important, on how much blood is ejected per beat; the amount of peripheral resistance is determined by the constriction or dilatation of the arteries.

The arteries in the vascular bed are dynamic and change size by constricting and dilating to control the supply of blood flow demanded by various parts of the body. Blood pressure must be maintained at a constant level and this is accomplished by reflexes in the cardiovascular system that alter the rate of flow as the size of the arterial beds varies.

LOW BLOOD PRESSURE

It is vital to the body that its blood pressure be maintained at an adequate level. The blood must be ejected from the heart with sufficient force to be transmitted to all the vascular beds that need a supply, most immediately and critically to the brain and heart itself. If the blood pressure falls suddenly and there is not enough blood to supply these vital organs, dangerously lowered blood pressure is present and the individual will become dizzy and possibly faint. Even more dangerous is the possibility that reduced blood flow to the heart may result in angina or a disturbance in the rhythm of the heart.

Blood pressure that is low enough to produce symptoms of this kind is usually seen only in physiologically abnormal situations, sometimes following a heart attack or in rare instances of severe blood loss when there is not enough blood to fill the vascular beds and the heart does not have enough blood to pump. This last situation is sometimes seen after an episode of bleeding from ulcers or following trauma such as a gunshot or stabbing wound that produces a severe loss of blood.

In these rare situations, it is essential that blood volume be restored at once if a significant amount has been lost. When there is not enough blood to maintain pressure, the patient may experience the serious symptoms of shock, a physiologic state quite different from marked emotional shock. Following a heart attack, the development of a markedly lowered blood pressure or hypotension can have ominous results. Drugs such as adrenalin or noradrenalin are used to constrict the systemic arteries and raise the blood pressure immediately.

Occasionally the loss of body fluids of any kind may decrease the blood pressure; people who have been sweating a great deal without adequate replacement of salt and water may become symptomatically hypotensive and faint. Another form of dangerously lowered blood pressure is neurogenic; an inappropriate firing of certain nerves leads to the dilatation or widening of the vascular space so that, even though cardiac output remains normal, the sudden increase in the volume of vessels drops the blood pressure. This promptly decreases the blood flow to the brain and produces symptoms of dizziness, often followed by fainting. Fainting spells seen in hysterical individuals or in those who are stressed by sudden emotional trauma are usually due to this mechanism.

In passing it should be noted that fainting has great survival value because when a normally upright human being falls down in a faint his head is made level with his heart. Since even the lowered blood pressure can then maintain blood flow to the brain, the best thing to do for a person who has fainted is to let him lie. Do not allow anyone to try to raise a person who has fainted into a sitting or standing position; allowing him to lie flat will in itself restore blood flow to the brain and allow a prompt recovery from the sudden condition that caused the faint.

Aside from these infrequent episodes, in most normal situations a low blood pressure is usually an asset because it places less strain on the heart and arteries. Usually only in situations of markedly depressed blood pressure, such as following an extreme loss of blood, does hypotension threaten the organism with shock. Only rarely will low blood pressure in an asymptomatic individual require medical attention.

NORMAL BLOOD PRESSURE

Normal levels of blood pressure are expressed in a range. That is, the "normal" systolic pressure (the upper figure) ranges from about 95 to 140 millimeters of mercury; the diastolic (lower figure) from 50 to 90. Many things, however, act to affect these so-called normal ranges and the proper level of blood pressure varies widely among individuals.

The patient's age has a great deal to do with his blood pressure levels, and the physician's choice of methods of management depends on many factors, including his assessment of the individual's ability to withstand the effects of high blood pressure. Some few individuals with moderately elevated blood pressure, who have no symptoms and in whom careful examination shows no damage to the target organs, may only be checked at frequent intervals.

The effect of age on blood pressure is seen most vividly in children who may have systolic blood pressures in the range of 60 to 70 mm of mercury—and have no symptoms. Young women can run systolic pressures of 90 to 95, shocklike levels in other people, and not have any symptoms of low blood pressure. If there are no symptoms and no evidence of insufficiency of blood flow to the organs, these lowered pressures are perfectly normal for some individuals.

The "upper" or systolic blood pressure that is measured during the ejection of blood from the heart can be elevated by any one of several factors. Anything that stiffens the walls of the arteries will increase the systolic blood pressure. If extensive atherosclerosis is present in the arteries, the arterial bed will be less elastic; the energy of the blood ejected from the heart, unable to stretch the walls, will instead raise the systolic blood pressure. A moderate amount of loss of elasticity of the arterial walls and atherosclerosis develops with aging, leading to the old rule of thumb that 100 added to a person's age will give the upper limit of normal blood pressure for him: a fifty-five-year-old man would have a normal upper limit of 155 according to this device. It should be noted that this is still only a range and there is no evidence that it is scientifically accurate; some investigators now feel that systolic blood pressure should not normally go up with aging.

There is also a dynamic cause for an increase in systolic pressure unrelated to age, which has to do with the amount of constriction in the arterial bed. Arterial constriction may be beneficial, acting to raise the blood pressure if it has fallen too low because of blood loss. In this instance vasoconstriction will decrease the vascular space and raise the pressure to the normal range.

Blood pressure levels are also related to the amount of blood flow, of course. In certain situations, if the heart puts out an increased amount of blood per stroke, the systolic blood pressure will rise as more blood is squeezed into a normal-sized vascular space. This is seen in patients, usually among the elderly, who have unusually slow heart rates, and in high output conditions such as hyperthyroidism, where the amount of blood put out by the heart per minute is increased. A slight rise in systolic blood pressure may also occur at the start of exercise when the heart must suddenly put out more blood.

In general, any blood pressure reading higher than 140 systolic or 90 diastolic (expressed as 140/90) warrants consideration of treatment of some kind. Again, it is the level of the blood pressure as well as the patient's response to the hypertension that will determine the kind of treatment and the vigor with which it is applied. As the blood pressure readings go up, of course, management becomes more imperative and more intense because the risk of a serious problem rises precipitously as the level becomes increasingly abnormal.

HIGH BLOOD PRESSURE

Long-term hypertension, the high blood pressure that leads to serious complications, is due to the chronic, inappropriate constriction of the arterial beds and a concomitant increase in peripheral resistance. This type of hypertension is expressed as a rise in the diastolic blood pressure to 90 mm of mercury and above. Any elevation in diastolic blood pressure, usually due to the constriction of arteries and arterioles in the vascular bed, is a serious matter that requires treatment, especially since it is usually accompanied by a rise in systolic pressure as well.

Blood pressure is normally controlled by a complex and sensitive system of feedback and response. Sensors in the cardiovascular system called baroreceptors are activated by changes in the arterial pressure. They alter the heart rate and the amount of blood ejected from the heart or the degree of vasoconstriction of the arteries in response to their reading of the body's blood pressure. Sensors act continuously to keep the blood pressure at a normal level if there are significant changes in blood volume or even a sudden change in posture from a prone to an upright position. Among people with hypertension, it is interesting that these baroreceptors appear to be set at a higher level than in normal people and it appears that high blood pressure is maintained in this way at constantly elevated levels.

Early in the development of hypertension the blood pressure may fluctuate widely, remaining in the normal range most of the time but rising to hypertensive levels at times of stress or excitement. For some people even the visit to the doctor's office—the physical examination and the actual measurement of the blood pressure itself—may produce elevated readings. In this case it is the fear of the diagnosis, rather than the determination itself, that alters the blood pressure level. Stress, anger, excitement, or even a cigarette or a cup of coffee can raise the blood pressure, but it is rare that an otherwise normal individual will have an elevation to a hypertensive level. That is, if a patient shows a rise high enough to be considered hypertension, especially in the diastolic pressure, the physician suspects that some abnormality may be present.

When abnormal blood pressure levels are detected at the initial examination, the physician will probably want to repeat the examination after some time has elapsed. If the blood pressure is found to be consistently elevated, or if the diastolic (lower figure) pressure is found, on even one examination, to be above 105 millimeters of mercury, therapy is indicated. Most physicians agree that a diastolic pressure of 115 and above should be immediately treated and carefully followed, for the evidence is clear that untreated hypertension at this level will produce cardiovascular and renal complications over a relatively short period of time. A recent study reported that people with chronically high diastolic pressure have an increased risk of developing heart disease, heart failure, stroke, or clinical kidney disease within a period of two to three years after the onset of hypertension.

If the blood pressure is never more than minimally elevated, remaining in the normal range most of the time, a change in the diet to effect weight reduction and a decrease in salt intake, along with some changes in the patient's mode of living to reduce habitual stress, may be enough to control the condition. If slightly more therapy is needed your physician may prescribe a mild sedative. What is important is that any elevation in blood pressure be followed carefully for several months so that appropriate therapy can be instituted at the earliest indication of more severe trouble.

LABILE HYPERTENSION

Blood pressure that bobs up and down between normal and abnormal levels is called *labile hypertension,* a condition that is confusing and troubling to the patient. He is told by one physician that he has high blood pressure only to be told a few weeks later that his pressure is perfectly normal. If the readings are done by two different physicians, as is so often the case in modern consultative medicine, rampant confusion may result in the patient's mind. The fact is that neither physician is incorrect or inaccurate in his blood pressure measurement, for in its early stages hypertension may appear and disappear sporadically. Patients with this kind of background should be seen frequently by their physicians and should have blood pressure determinations repeated at regular intervals. Labile hypertension, or any transient mild rise in blood pressure, may signal impending fixed hypertension; because of its widespread effects and possible complications, this more serious form should be watched for with vigilance.

Because everyone wants to believe that everything is just fine, most people will remember normal blood pressure readings and not even think about the periods when it might be elevated. This is extremely unwise: labile hypertension, with its periods of high blood pressure, is an unmistakable sign of trouble and to deny its presence is counterproductive and dangerous. Therapy directed toward labile hypertension moderates the peaks and rises and, although without therapy the blood pressure may be normal for periods of time, treatment effectively reduces the damage done to the target organs by episodes of markedly elevated blood pressure. Long-term therapy is continued, usually in moderated amounts, to eliminate the periods of abnormal elevation.

HOW HYPERTENSION AFFECTS THE BODY

The treatment of hypertension is truly preventive medicine. Except to alleviate the dizziness and headaches experienced by some few patients when their blood pressure is elevated, the reduction of abnormally elevated blood pressure is directed toward preventing damage to the target organs—the heart, brain, kidneys, and blood vessels.

A continuously elevated blood pressure is especially harmful to the heart. In the presence of hypertension the heart must pump the blood with a greater than normal force to overcome the resistance in the constricted arteries. This added work load on the heart causes the left ventricle to enlarge and its muscle walls to hypertrophy or thicken. After a period of time the left ventricle is no longer able to tolerate the increased work load and the heart begins to fail. The heart increases in size and any exertion is accompanied by shortness of breath. Over a period of years, the heart gradually becomes more and more impaired, its failure more pronounced, until normal activity cannot be tolerated. Data from the Framingham study, in which a large population was followed for more than fifteen years, suggest that hypertensive heart disease evolving in this way is the most common cause of congestive heart failure, surpassing both coronary artery disease and rheumatic heart disease in frequency.

The increase in the work load of the heart and the hypertrophy of its walls caused by chronically elevated blood pressure increase the amount of oxygen needed by the heart to function; coronary blood flow must be stepped up to supply this demand. If there is an area of narrowing in a coronary vessel due to coronary occlusion, the need for more blood flow may not be met and symptoms of starvation, or ischemia, will result. For this reason, the pains of angina pectoris are frequently seeen in patients with hypertension who also have coronary artery disease. Alleviation of hypertension in such patients commonly relieves this angina, allowing them to exercise without pain to a degreee that was not possible while the blood pressure was elevated.

Elevated blood pressure also causes significant disease in the vascular system. Because the heart ejects blood with increased force, the arteries are repeatedly traumatized. If part of the arterial wall has been weakened by a congenital abnormality or by the presence of atherosclerosis, the increased force of the blood may cause this area to rupture and bleed. For this reason severe nosebleeds are often a sign of elevated blood pressure, and bleeding of the type that is due to hypertension can be catastrophic if the vessel involved is in the brain. A hemorrhagic stroke then occurs and this is one of the mechanisms by which high blood pressure can paralyze.

The prolonged stress of hypertension on arterial walls can also lead to the development of aneurysms or "blowouts," either in the aorta or in a peripheral artery. Aneurysms occur in an area of vessel that is weakened; constant high blood pressure causes the weakened area to balloon out through a sequence not very different from that which takes place when an inner tube is filled with more air than it can hold. Any weakened area bulges under the strain and the stretched walls become dangerously thin. The continued pounding of increased blood pressure may cause the aneurysm to rupture, producing a very serious consequence of high blood pressure. Aneurysms of all parts of the arterial system are rare in general but more common in people with hypertension.

Other serious vascular problems can be traced to the increased mechanical pressure of hypertension. In addition to ruptured vessels and the possibility of developing aneurysms, the blood vessels may respond to the injury of persistent high pressure with scarring and thickening of the vessel walls, a process which narrows the vessel opening. This serious effect of hypertension is especially destructive when it occurs in the kidneys or brain. Longstanding hypertension, which can be caused by kidney disease, can itself narrow the arteries within the kidneys so extensively that renal insufficiency and life-threatening uremia may result. Continued hypertension over many years can also cause chronic changes in the vessels of the brain and the loss of certain brain functions. Mental deterioration and confusion may result if high blood pressure is not controlled by medication or other means.

HYPERTENSION AND ATHEROSCLEROSIS

Hypertension is one of the three most important risk factors associated with the development of coronary artery disease, high cholesterol levels and cigarette smoking being the only others that approach it in prevalence or seriousness. Although it is not entirely clear exactly how hypertension predisposes to atherosclerosis, there are a number of theories to explain the relationship. The ultrafiltration theory of the development of atherosclerosis suggests that serum is pushed by the force of the blood pressure through the inner lining of the vessel walls to become embedded within the wall. All of the constituents of the serum except cholesterol and other lipids are removed by the body's normal defense mechanism. The cholesterol remains in the wall and accumulates to form an atherosclerotic plaque. According to this theory, since the blood pressure within the vessel is higher than normal, there is a greater tendency for the serum to be pushed into its wall and the development of atherosclerosis is thus enhanced.

Another theory put forth to explain the higher incidence of atherosclerotic heart disease among hypertensives relates to the increased turbulence in the vascular tree caused by the force of the high blood pressure. It has been noted in a number of studies that much of the atherosclerosis in coronary arteries occurs at areas of bending or branching where the turbulence of the blood flow would be increased. The mechanical force of the turbulence may damage the *intima,* the inside layer of the vessel, making it more permeable to the filtration of serum and the cholesterol it contains, leading again to the formation of plaque. Such intimal damage may also stimulate wall muscle cells to react abnormally, absorbing cholesterol and lipid material.

Increased turbulence may also traumatize the blood and lead to the formation of small platelet clots on the inside surface of the vessel. One theory holds that these small clots damage the vessel wall in a way that makes it more permeable to ultrafiltration. Or the clots themselves may serve as the nidus for the development of an atherosclerotic plaque. The presence of a small intra-arterial clot may be the initial insult that goes on to become an atherosclerotic plaque. Recent data have suggested that platelet clots on the endothelial surface of the intima may directly stimulate muscle cells in the vessel wall to absorb lipids and cholesterol and eventually lead to the development of an atherosclerotic plaque. Since clots forming in the arteries of the brain because of the increased turbulence associated with hypertension may lead to the development of a thrombotic stroke, the more common form of cerebrovascular accident, this mechanism may account for the high incidence of stroke among patients with hypertension.

HYPERTENSIVE CRISIS

Another serious complication of hypertension is a sudden marked rise in blood pressure to a diastolic level above 150 millimeters of mercury. Termed a hypertensive crisis, this is an uncommon medical emergency. Manifested by severe headaches, dizziness, vomiting, and frequently severe chest pain and heart failure, these acute episodes sometimes culminate in convulsions and other signs of compromise of the central nervous system. Fortunately, lowering the blood pressure at once with effective medication usually reverses the condition promptly; untreated crises can cause strokes and sudden death.

AVOIDING THE COMPLICATIONS OF HYPERTENSION

This necessarily brief review of the consequences of long-term hypertension can end on an optimistic note, for there is no question that treatment does make a difference. In a well-controlled, carefully documented study of high blood pressure among patients in a Veterans Administration hospital, it was found that men with markedly elevated diastolic pressures, above 115 millimeters of mercury, who were not treated had a much greater incidence of illness than a matched group who had been successfully treated to lower blood pressure levels within normal ranges. The same results were seen in a group whose overall blood pressure was lower, although still in the abnormal range of 105 to 115 diastolic; those who were not treated had far more of the complications of hypertension than those whose blood pressure was under medical control. Although the differences were not so striking in this latter group, the study left little doubt that untreated hypertension carries with it a risk of significant danger to the heart, the brain, and the kidneys. Since the effects of high blood pressure are reversible and since even slight elevations can be treated successfully, there is no longer any question that all hypertension must be controlled.

ESSENTIAL HYPERTENSION

Although the diagnosis, complications, and effects of hypertension have been well defined, the actual cause of hypertension is even now only partially understood. Except for a small percentage of patients who have one of a few specific etiologies described in detail below, the vast majority of hypertensive patients are considered to have what is called *essential hypertension* or high blood pressure of no specific cause. The American Medical Association estimates that 90 percent of all people with high blood pressure have essential hypertension that cannot be accounted for by any underlying disorder.

A "wastebasket" term, used to describe the still unfathomed causes of most high blood pressure, essential hypertension is the subject of a great deal of research effort in laboratories all over the world. Although the cause of essential hypertension is not fully understood, we can derive some knowledge from more specifically known types of high blood pressure. Thus, from an early animal model of hypertension developed by Dr. H. Goldblatt in the 1930s, we have considerable knowledge of the important relationship between the kidneys and high blood pressure in man. Goldblatt reasoned that, since many hypertensive patients also had kidney disease, it was reasonable to suspect some sort of cause and effect relationship. By narrowing one of the renal arteries and compromising the blood flow to one kidney in a number of experimental animals, Goldblatt was able to produce elevated blood pressures. This pioneering work has been replicated many times in experimental animals and correlates have been documented in human studies.

The relationship of blood flow to the kidneys and blood pressure is central to the proper functioning of the human body. Although an apparent function of the kidneys is to rid the body of the toxic wastes of metabolism, their more fundamental role is to maintain the salt and water balance of the body. The kidneys act as the fine tuning apparatus to maintain the amount of fluid in the vascular spaces needed for life, no more and no less. This vital balance is achieved by means of a complex action of feedback and response that is exquisitely sensitive.

Greatly simplified, the kidneys regulate the body's fluid volume through a system of especially structured capillaries and tubules that are able to selectively retain or excrete salt and water in response to a number of stimuli. These stimuli include intravascular fluid volume, the concentration of salts in the blood, the hormonal environment, and the blood pressure. Through certain specialized blood vessels, the kidneys can sense the blood pressure and judge the amount of volume coming to them. If for some reason the kidneys sense that not enough blood is flowing to them, they respond as though the reason for the inadequate flow is that blood pressure and blood volume are inadequate. The kidneys signal the rest of the body to conserve or increase the blood volume and to increase the blood pressure by constricting arteries throughout the system.

This response has a high survival value because, if there is no obstruction in the renal arteries, a decrease in kidney flow is most often caused by blood loss, followed by a significant decrease in blood volume and the almost certain occurrence of shock. Increasing the blood pressure in this way would be lifesaving, for example, following a serious wound or bleeding injury of any kind. When the kidneys sense that blood flow coming to them may be inadequate for their needs, they interpret this to mean that blood flow is compromised throughout the body; they act at once to raise the systemic blood pressure and the amount of volume in the vascular space.

It is only in the last ten to fifteen years that the biochemical mechanism for this intriguing response has been understood. Low renal blood flow activates specialized kidney cells to produce a substance called *renin*. Renin converts *angiotensinogen,* a compound produced by the liver, from its usual inactive form to the active form called *angiotensin*. Angiotensin has two effects. First, it raises the blood pressure by constricting the arteries. In addition, it causes the adrenal gland to put out a steroid hormone called *aldosterone* which causes the kidney to retain salt and water in the body, thereby increasing the intravascular blood volume.

This sequence occurs normally in everyone, constantly, as the body works ceaselessly to function effectively and maintain its integrity. The feedback mechanism senses when flow to the kidneys is sufficient; the kidneys stop putting out renin, the production of angiotensin stops, and the secretion of salt-retaining hormones from the adrenal gland comes to an end. In certain situations, however, the system may trigger or continue its operation inappropriately. The body does not respond to the increase in blood volume by shutting down renin production, the normal feedback mechanism is somehow impaired, and the continued stimulation produces hypertension.

Although most patients with hypertension do not have obvious abnormalities in the blood flow to their kidneys, it is interesting that many people with what has been previously considered to be essential hypertension are found to have inappropriately increased renin levels. Moreover, the high renin levels in these individuals are correlated with the development of the complications of hypertension; the higher the renin level, the more frequent or widespread the deleterious results. This work is relatively recent, has yet to be confirmed by studies that replicate its findings, and has been questioned by other investigators, but it does suggest an exciting new rationale of treatment for hypertension where the vigor of the therapy would depend on the renin levels.

"CURABLE" HYPERTENSION

Although most hypertensive patients have no apparent cause for their high blood pressure—essential hypertension—there are a few specific abnormalities that can be cured with surgery or other means. For this reason most physicians, on discovering hypertension, will do a "work-up" to rule out these specific remediable causes before they start therapy for essential hypertension or if the patient does not respond readily to attempts to control the blood pressure.

The doctor will look first to the kidneys for a specific cause of high blood pressure. If a localized area of atherosclerosis narrows one of the arteries feeding the kidneys, they will respond to the threat of reduced blood flow by secreting high levels of renin and the aldosterone-angiotensin system will be activated causing hypertension. In order to determine whether a patient's high blood pressure is caused by some obstruction in the renal artery, an intravenous pyelogram (IVP) is done. X-ray films are taken of the kidneys after a radio-opaque dye has been injected; the speed with which the two kidneys opacify allows inferences to be made about the presence or absence of an obstructive lesion in one of the arteries. If the IVP suggests an obstructive lesion, further studies may be done by arteriography to get a better picture of the vasculature feeding the kidneys.

Once the actual position of the obstruction is visualized, surgery can be considered. The narrowed area of the artery can be surgically removed and the artery reconnected to provide unimpeded blood flow to the kidneys, curing the hypertension in many cases. When the unimpeded blood flow is normal, the stimulus for the secretion of renin is halted, and in many cases as the renin levels drop the blood pressure comes down significantly.

A rare kidney tumor which causes hypertension may be picked up during a routine examination for persistent high blood pressure. The tumor may press on the blood vessels in one of the kidneys, activating the renin-angiotensin system. The IVP usually discloses a tumor of this kind, and its surgical removal may cure the hypertension it produces.

Hypertension is infrequently caused by tumors in or overactivity of parts of the adrenal gland. Each of these types of tumors causes hypertension by increasing the secretions of substances that raise the blood pressure. If the tumor occurs in the cells that produce adrenalin or noradrenalin, a tumor known technically as a *pheochromocytoma*, the blood pressure is elevated because the effects of the sympathetic nervous system are simulated.

Tumors of the cells of the adrenal gland that produce cortisone can cause hypertension. The physician may suspect the presence of this disease, known technically as Cushing's syndrome, when he notices some characteristic changes in the body fat distribution, hair patterns, skin lesions, and specific bone problems.

A tumor or hyperplasia (benign overgrowth) of cells in the parts of the adrenal gland that produces aldosterone (the hormone that causes the kidney to retain salt) can also produce hypertension in a condition known as Conn's syndrome. These tumors are diagnosed by measuring the amounts of the substances secreted by the tumor in a twenty-four-hour urine specimen. Because aldosterone causes the excretion of large amounts of potassium as it retains sodium, an aldosterone-producing tumor is suspected when excessive amounts of potassium are found in the urine and reduced amounts in the blood. Most adrenal tumors are noncancerous and surgery can be curative. Adrenal hyperplasia frequently responds to medical therapy to control the mild hypertension and surgery may not be needed.

Very rarely a tumor of the *parathyroids*, the glands which produce the hormone that regulates calcium balance in the body, can cause mild hypertension. Diagnosis is made by measuring calcium levels in the blood and removal of the tumor in most cases cures this form of hypertension.

A rare mechanical problem, the congenital narrowing of a

portion of the aorta known as a coarctation, is another cause of high blood pressure that can be surgically corrected.

Although these surgical advances are truly remarkable in their effect, only a very small percentage of hypertensive patients can be treated surgically. In most medical centers, unless there is evidence of a tumor, only the severely hypertensive patient who does not respond medically is considered for surgery. The decision to operate is influenced by the patient's response to medical treatment, the physician's judgment of the situation, and the local practices with regard to renal vascular surgery. In some centers, however, excellent results have been obtained and surgery of this kind frees the patient from lifelong medical treatment for hypertension.

KIDNEY DISEASE AND HYPERTENSION

Some forms of kidney disease lead to both renal failure and the development of hypertension. The finding of high blood pressure may draw the doctor's attention to these diseases, leading to immediate measures to halt their progression.

Chronic infections of the kidneys, for example, often starting as isolated bouts of acute infection, will cause the loss of more and more kidney substance. If the vasculature is also involved there is an inappropriate secretion of renin, with all of its effects on blood volume and the development of hypertension. For this reason, as is stressed in the discussion of heart disease in women, even minor urinary tract infections should be considered seriously and treated vigorously.

In men, conditions of the prostate gland may obstruct the bladder outflow tract and make it difficult to excrete urine. If the bladder remains enlarged because it cannot empty properly, there may be reflux back through the ureters and into both kidneys. If this goes on for a long period of time, renal damage and hypertension may result. Incomplete emptying of the bladder also predisposes to infection in the bladder and kidneys and can lead to renal impairment and high blood pressure in this way. Surgical relief of the prostate obstruction will usually reverse the progression of the kidney involvement, and if done early enough may ameliorate the hypertension.

The formation of stones in the urinary tract, the kidneys, ureters, or bladder can also cause obstruction and its sequelae:

infection, kidney damage, and occasionally hypertension. Stones can form because of the presence of infection in the urine, but are frequently caused by an underlying metabolic abnormality, such as high calcium (hyperparathyroidism) or high uric acid (gout) levels in the blood.

Another disease that can lead to kidney failure, especially in the rare finding of hypertension in children, is glomerulonephritis. It is most commonly preceded by a streptococcal infection, often the common "strep" throat of children, or in some cases by a skin infection caused by streptococcus. Strep infections of this kind are also often followed by rheumatic fever. In most cases glomerulonephritis is an acute and self-limiting disease, but it can go into a subacute phase and recur in chronic form. This is an uncommon cause of hypertension in the adult but, since it can lead to kidney problems and the high blood pressure associated with them, the development of glomerulonephritis in children should be prevented by the vigorous treatment of any recognized strep infection.

Any systemic condition or disease that leads to a loss of kidney substance can eventually produce renal insufficiency, a life-threatening situation where the kidneys are unable to function adequately and the wastes they must excrete back up, causing the condition known as uremia. A serious toxic condition, uremia will cause death if vigorous treatment including dialysis, artificial kidney treatments, or transplant is not begun at once. Hypertension is usually seen well before severe irreversible renal insufficiency develops and can act as a warning signal to call attention to these serious underlying diseases.

DRUG-INDUCED HYPERTENSION

Hypertension can also be caused by some few drugs taken for other reasons, so long-term therapy should never be undertaken until any medication that might cause the condition is discontinued, at least temporarily.

Perhaps the most widely used drug predisposing to hypertension is the contraceptive pill. Although it is a rare complication of the pill—only about one percent of the vast numbers of women on the pill appear to develop hypertension—its widespread use makes the oral contraceptive agent one of the major causes of hypertension among women.

For this reason women with a history of high blood pressure should avoid the contraceptive pill, and all women should see their physician regularly for blood pressure determinations while on it. If hypertension should appear, the pill must be discontinued at once. Blood pressure sometimes remains elevated for several months after the contraceptive pills have been stopped but, if the condition persists longer than this, an evaluation should be done to rule out other possible causes of high blood pressure. Women with a personal or family history of heart disease or circulatory problems of any kind should be carefully evaluated before being placed on the pill.

Another class of drugs that almost invariably leads to blood pressure elevations are those that mimic the effects of the sympathetic nervous system. These include the amphetamines, dexedrine, benzedrine, methedrine ("speed"), and combinations of these drugs with barbiturates (Dexamyl®). These are drugs of abuse and anyone embarking on their long-term use should consider the consequences carefully. Their action is similar to that of adrenalin, accelerating the heart rate, increasing the strength of contraction of the heart, constricting the arteriolar bed, and elevating the blood pressure. Drugs of this kind create a nervous kind of "high," accompanied by palpitations and a type of exhilaration that some people find exciting. Used illegally for "kicks," or by some misguided people for purposes of weight reduction, these drugs produce an agitated kind of heightened energy that is always followed by an inordinate sense of fatigue and letdown.

Stimulant drugs of this kind, "uppers," are extremely dangerous and should never be taken recklessly or without the careful supervision of a physician for some few rare conditions. By speeding the metabolism and increasing the work of the heart, they create a situation of great potential hazard. Anyone with even slightly elevated blood pressure runs the risk of blowing out a vessel in the brain and thus suffering a stroke as a result of the sudden acceleration of blood pressure produced by these drugs. In people with coronary artery disease this stimulation can lead to angina and the possible occurrence of an infarction. Patients with any form of underlying heart disease can be thrown into heart failure, and even those with minimal heart problems can experience arrthymias after taking stimulant drugs.

A rare disease of the renal arteries is a generalized fibrosis of the back wall of the abdominal cavity. The area is severely scarred and the arteries which must pass through them are narrowed as a consequence. Some drugs are suspected of causing this fibrosis, among them phenacetin—often present in headache remedies sold over the counter. If you use such remedies often, you should read the label carefully and switch to something that does not contain phenacetin. Although this finding is by no means conclusive— again coincidence may be the ultimate cause—if nonphenacetin products are available it might be prudent to use them instead for long-term conditions.

HYPERTENSION AND THE TOXEMIA OF PREGNANCY

During the reproductive years, women are subject to a serious complication of pregnancy called eclampsia, or toxemia. (The hypertension which is characteristic of toxemia is discussed in detail in Volume II.) Some women who experience toxemia may go on to have sustained hypertension, but in most cases the blood pressure levels return to normal when the pregnancy is concluded. Women who have hypertension prior to pregnancy have an increased risk of toxemia, and they should be watched carefully. After one bout of toxemia there is a slightly increased risk during subsequent pregnancies. Good prenatal care is necessary, and blood pressure must be checked frequently, especially during the last months of pregnancy.

"TREATABLE" HYPERTENSION

Although I have pointed out those few forms of hypertension that are known to have a specific cause, including those that can be treated surgically, it should be emphasized that the vast majority of people with high blood pressure—estimates range from 80 percent to 90 percent—fit into none of these disease categories and are considered to have essential hypertension, elevated blood pressure with no known specific cause. On examination they are found to have normal laboratory and x-ray findings, and a thorough work-up discloses no specific cause for a chronically elevated blood pressure level. What is the cause of high blood pressure in patients of this kind? Frankly, no one knows and the useful term "essential hypertension" will remain until more work has been done on the etiology or causation of high blood pressure.

As research proceeds, it may be that more of the patients now classified as essential hypertensives will be found to have some specific cause for their high blood pressure. Preliminary work done recently at Columbia University has suggested that, even in the absence of demonstrable kidney disease, many people with essential hypertension have inappropriately elevated renin levels. And the presence of high renin is associated with the complications of hypertension to a significant degree, damage to the target organs in the form of coronary atherosclerosis, heart attacks, and stroke increasing in these patients as the renin levels go up. These patients also have a higher incidence of neurological problems and an earlier development of kidney failure.

Since these data represent the results of only a few studies, it is too early to draw any conclusions from this work. Subsequent research may indicate, however, that patients with essential hypertension characterized by high renin levels should be treated vigorously to avoid the complications and consequences of long-term hypertension, whereas those with proven low renin levels may not need intensive or prolonged therapy. The value of this work may be its suggestion that the answer to the riddle of essential hypertension in many patients may lie within what appear to be normal kidneys and their renin-angiotensin-aldosterone system.

Another recent study of a group of patients with essential hypertension disclosed that many had high levels of circulating serum noradrenalin and adrenalin. These levels were not high enough to suggest the presence of a tumor, but there was an indication of inappropriate activity of the sympathetic nervous system, another clue to one of the causes of essential hypertension.

It is heartening, however, that, regardless of the reason for the essential hypertension, lowering the blood pressure to normal levels will reduce the risk of cardiovascular complications. The natural history of hypertension is that untreated high blood pressure continues to rise over a period of time and, depending upon the ability of the body to withstand its damaging assaults, progressively attacks the target organs—the heart, the brain, and the kidneys—and can eventually lead to premature death. Since men seem to suffer these effects more frequently than women, high blood pressure must be treated more vigorously in men.

Once hypertension is diagnosed it is necessary that patients be treated throughout their lifetime if they are to avoid its almost inevitable consequences. This does not mean that treatment is always at a maximum, for in most cases once the hypertension is brought under control the dosage schedule can be maintained at a moderate level. But one of the great difficulties of long-term treatment of this kind is that it is only human nature to want to abandon treatment altogether once the first beneficial effect has been achieved. The average patient is delighted to forget the entire episode as soon as he feels better and the blood pressure reading comes down to near normal levels. Every physician has records of patients who were treated for hypertension and disappeared, only to surface again years later with serious problems that could have been avoided by continued treatment.

Fortunately, hypertension can be successfully treated with a progression of gradually more potent modalities, starting with measures that can be instituted by the patient himself and ranging up through drugs that vary in power as well as in specific effects. The treatment modality chosen depends on the severity of the condition and on the likelihood of damage to the target organs; the success of any measure, of course, depends on the cooperation of the patient and his willingness to participate in the management of his condition.

THE "HYPERTENSIVE" PERSONALITY

The first, simplest, and in many cases most effective treatment for hypertension is some expertise in the simple art of relaxation. When a human being encounters a stressful situation, whether it is a life-threatening event like a genuine emergency or an extremely irritating encounter with another person, the sympathetic nervous system is activated and the blood pressure rises. In normal people the rise in blood pressure is modest and rarely reaches abnormal levels. But hypertensive individuals, especially those with the early form known as labile hypertension, react to stress with marked elevations of the blood pressure.

Although it may be appropriate to respond to genuine stress

with a violent physiologic outpouring—when your life is threatened you need the increased blood pressure to respond quickly—people with hypertensive personalities seem to evoke this major response for relatively minor annoyances. Whether the type of personality that overreacts to minor emotional trauma really "causes" hypertension is as yet unsettled, but it is evident that avoiding such situations altogether, or learning to take them in stride, is quite effective in reducing high blood pressure levels.

Before the potent therapeutic antihypertensive drugs were available, rest and frequent vacations were routinely prescribed as the principal treatment for hypertension. In an insightful case study reported in the prestigious *Annals of Internal Medicine,* the details of the management of President Franklin D. Roosevelt's hypertension were revealed for the first time, twenty-five years after the day of his death. In the 1930s, when Roosevelt evidenced dangerously high blood pressure levels, his physicians prescribed the treatment then available: mild sedation, dietary management, and, most important, frequent rest periods away from Washington. The president was maintained in this way for many years with only minimal symptoms. Rest alone is usually not enough to alleviate all traces of hypertension and at that time inadequate control of hypertension could only delay the appearance of the serious consequences of long-term high blood pressure. The president was to die of a stroke in 1945, some years after the onset of his condition, but there is no question that proper living habits and relaxation materially aided in his management.

Learning to respond appropriately to stress of varying magnitudes is not easy; it involves a great deal of soul-searching and discipline. Stress and the hypertension associated with it are major risk factors in the development of coronary atherosclerosis; its pathophysiology and suggestions for dealing with stress are described in Chapter 7.

Further evidence of the link between the mind or the emotions and the level of blood pressure comes from interesting new research being conducted at Rockefeller University and elsewhere. In these studies subjects are given sensing devices and trained to raise or lower their blood pressure at will. More work remains to be done, since in most cases the results are not permanent, but research of this kind points to a new technique for the treatment of hypertension. The control of blood pressure levels and other autonomic bodily responses were previously thought to be beyond the control of the conscious mind, so these findings open up a new and intriguing research horizon.

There have also been reports that Yoga and other forms of mind control have been effective in lowering the blood pressure. As this is written there are studies in the popular press as well as in the medical literature reporting good results in lowering blood pressure by means of Transcendental Meditation. Subjects practicing Transcendental Meditation regularly were able to achieve a relaxation response that in some patients lowered blood pressure about 10 to 15 percent. It is difficult to assess the results in many of the reports I have seen, but anything that helps to control hypertension should certainly be investigated further.

I would caution, however, that no one with existing hypertension abandon dietary or drug regimens while experimenting with this relatively untried method of control unless he is under the supervision of an investigator who is a physician and is part of a recognized research study. While it may be true that the conscious mind can be trained to exert a beneficial effect, it is also true that hypertension is too serious and complex a condition to warrant the discontinuance of methods that have proved effective.

One of the simplest ways to avoid an inappropriate response to minor stress is to always face the problems of the day after a good night's sleep. For patients who are tense and nervous, and for those with any tendency toward high blood pressure, eight to ten hours of rest at night—in bed, in the dark, whether asleep or not —will go a long way toward tempering the strains of the day.

THE DIETARY CONTROL OF HYPERTENSION

Dietary control plays another simple but significant role in the management of high blood pressure. Most important, obesity itself appears to predispose to the development of hypertension in some people. Hypertensive patients who are overweight can frequently bring their blood pressure levels down just by losing weight. Sometimes a judicious weight loss will be enough to put the blood pressure levels into the normal ranges, in this way avoiding drug treatment. Weight control and some methods for its successful attainment are described at length in Chapter 9.

Even people without a weight problem can alter their diet to decrease the amount of salt they eat, a simple measure that often reduces high blood pressure levels. One of the earliest recognized therapies for severe hypertension, developed in the 1930s when patients with severe and rapidly progressive hypertension could expect to live only a few years, was a diet that contained absolutely no salt and consisted mainly of rice and fruit. Poorly nourishing and difficult to live with, this extreme diet is not necessary today because of the truly outstanding drugs that are available to treat even the most resistant forms of hypertension. However, experiences derived from the use of very rigorously salt-free diet in the management of hypertensive patients proved that salt reduction is effective, and a less severe reduction in salt intake is now more common and has been shown to be a useful adjunct to therapy of any kind.

So, unless your doctor prescribes a strictly salt-free diet, you can easily adhere to a reasonable diet that limits salt effectively. All of the obviously salty foods should be avoided; most of them are of the snack variety, extremely high in calories, and probably do not belong in anyone's diet. These include potato chips, pretzels, olives, popcorn, salted nuts, and highly seasoned snack crackers. All foods that are salted or smoked should be avoided: bologna, hot dogs, delicatessen meats and fishes, herring, and the like. Pickled meats, fishes, and vegetables such as cucumbers should not be eaten because they are prepared in brine, a strong salt solution. Most canned soups are rather highly salted and a good salt-free diet should probably substitute homemade varieties that can be seasoned in other ways. If no salt is added at the table, this minimally restricted diet will markedly decrease salt intake.

Another tip to people seeking to reduce their salt intake, both because of high blood pressure or the demands of pregnancy: remedies for heartburn and indigestion sold over the counter, especially the seltzer types, are extremely high in sodium. They will increase the salt intake significantly and should not be used.

This moderate type of low salt diet, usually effective in lowering the blood pressure, is not so extreme that any additional use of drugs will lead to excessive salt depletion. If circumstances require that salt intake be limited even further, your physician will provide sound advice and more specific instruction.

HYPERTENSION AND SMOKING

Another measure that is effective in reducing blood pressure levels is to stop smoking. Inhaling tobacco and nicotine stimulates the sympathetic nervous system and produces the jolt that makes smoking enjoyable. But increased sympathetic activity acutely raises the blood pressure, and in hypertensives this effect may be prolonged. Smoking is not a habit that is easily given up but since it is also an important risk factor in the development of coronary artery disease, specific methods for its control are suggested in Chapter 8.

THE PHARMACOLOGIC CONTROL OF HYPERTENSION

Essential hypertension that cannot be controlled by dietary manipulation, salt reduction, or by changes in living habits must be treated medically. Fortunately, the drugs that are available today can be considered among the genuine advances of modern medicine. Of six distinct families or types, these drugs can be used to control almost every form of high blood pressure.

In patients with mild hypertension, moderate sedation will sometimes produce a significant decrease in blood pressure. Phenobarbital, for example, or one of the mild tranquilizers may often relax the individual enough to bring his pressure down. Coupled with some insight into living habits and some tempering of the patient's reaction to stress, this is often quite an effective method of hypertension control. The only side effect of these drugs is the drowsiness that sometimes accompanies them at the start of therapy, but after taking them for a short time the drowsiness disappears and general relaxation replaces it. Sedation alone can drop the diastolic pressure five to ten points in some patients and is especially effective in the control of labile hypertension.

Another useful class of drugs, of rather recent development, is the oral diuretics. Taken one to three times a day, thiazide or similar types of diuretic drugs are a genuine advance in the treatment of hypertension. Since they act to increase the salt and water output, they are often used in the treatment of salt retention states such as congestive heart failure. Hypertensives who tend to retain fluid and who have edema and swelling of the legs and ankles often note rapid relief as these drugs increase the amount of urination and step up the loss of fluids. (This is usually noted during the first few days of treatment; after that there is only a slight increase in the amount of urination.)

Diuretics affect the blood pressure in two ways. Early in therapy there is a decrease in the amount of intravascular blood volume; with less blood in the vascular space the blood pressure goes down. Within a few months, however, blood volume returns to near normal ranges. It is then that the other diuretic effect, not so clearly documented, appears to take over. By depleting the sodium contained in the walls of the vasculature, diuretics reduce the tendency toward vasoconstriction. This effect also appears to moderate the body's response to the always present stimuli of the sympathetic nervous system.

Diuretic drugs are frequently used alone, but any drug regimen beyond simple sedation usually includes a diuretic agent because diuretics seem to potentiate or increase the action of any other drug that is administered, allowing some reduction in the dosage of other antihypertensive drugs. And a lower dose of a number of drugs, rather than a high dose of a single drug, reduces the chances of significant side effects.

Every pharmacologic agent that is effective has side effects of some kind; medicine is essentially the art of balancing side effects against the possible benefits of a drug. Fortunately, the side effects of diuretics are minor, are usually part of their action, and in most cases do not cause the discontinuance of the drug.

The loss of potassium is the principal side effect of the diuretics. This loss is usually mild and is easily managed by the simple expedient of always taking the drug with a glass of fruit juice. Most fruits contain potassium and taking the drug in this way helps guard against the possible development of a low potassium state. Other potassium-rich foods include tomatoes (raw and in juice form), potatoes, bananas, cantaloupe, dates, buttermilk, almonds, cashews and peanuts, baked beans, cooked greens, and nearly all raw vegetables.

Potassium replacement is especially important for patients on high doses of diuretic drugs and for those who are also taking digitalis in any of its forms (digoxin, digitoxin) because a low serum level of potassium can lower the threshold for the development of toxicity. In most cases a substantial amount of food containing potassium is sufficient to avoid this situation and when necessary the physician can prescribe a potassium supplement, usually in liquid form.

Thus when your physician tells you to take diuretic pills with a glass of orange juice he is practicing good preventive medicine along with good nutrition. If potassium is not replaced, an occasional patient may develop symptoms of muscle weakness and lethargy. This occurs only rarely and can be treated effectively with supplemental potassium. Apart from this occasional side effect, the oral diuretic drugs have proved their efficacy and effectiveness consistently and have become a mainstay of today's antihypertensive therapy.

Another class of drugs used to treat hypertension works by manipulating the sympathetic nervous system and its neurotransmitters. You will recall that the sympathetic nervous system is the system that is activated in an emergency to prepare the body for fight or flight. Its chemical neurotransmitters, adrenalin and noradrenalin, act to increase the heart rate, the strength of the heart's contraction, and the blood pressure.

Many patients with essential hypertension appear to have either an overresponsiveness or an overactivity of the sympathetic nervous system. By blocking these effects pharmacologically, especially the vasoconstrictive effects that elevate the blood pressure, hypertension can be reduced. These sympathetic blocking agents tend to either blunt the effect of the neurotransmitter by blocking its site of action or deplete the body of these substances by interfering with their storage.

It is interesting, and further evidence of the connection between high blood pressure and the emotions, that reserpine, one of the major drugs of this class, has been used for centuries in India for the treatment of psychiatric disorders. Derived from the rauwolfia plant, reserpine was brought from herbal medicine to the West in the late 1940s as one of the first tranquilizing agents. Effective in the treatment of mild to moderately severe hypertension, reserpine counters the effects of the sympathetic nervous system by reducing the amount of epinephrine and norepinephrine present in the body. Depleting the catecholamines in this way reduces the reactivity of the arterial vascular system and causes a drop in blood pressure.

This effective drug is used orally over long periods of time and parenterally, by injection, in patients with acutely high levels of blood pressure. Its side effects are few, ranging from stuffiness in the nose to an occasional case of diarrhea. A rare patient may experience some heartburn, and reserpine will occasionally increase the symptoms of an ulcer. If a patient has had an ulcer, it is important that he inform his doctor before any antihypertensive treatment is begun.

Sometimes the psychotropic effects of the drug may cause an occasional complaint of bad dreams, feelings of depression, and difficulty in falling asleep, although in many cases the patient will report an increased sense of well-being.

Aldomet® (alpha-methyldopa) is another drug that works on the sympathetic nervous system. Unlike reserpine, however, it does not deplete the body of catecholamines but instead acts as a false adrenalin and noradrenalin, replacing these substances in the nerve endings. When the nerve is stimulated the false transmitter is released and the sympathetic nervous system is knocked out as the ineffective impostor replaces the normal neurotransmitter. This is ingenious drug manipulation and the alpha-methyldopa drug is effective. They have few side effects and can be given in varied doses as required. Aldomet is usually given, along with a thiazide diuretic, three or four times a day in amounts that are determined by the severity of the hypertension.

Guanethidine, or Ismelin®, is a potent agent that is used in the treatment of severe or moderately severe hypertension. This drug also acts to block the effects of epinephrine and norepinephrine release near the nerve endings of the vessels, in this way inhibiting the vasoconstrictive effects of sympathetic stimulation. These are effective drugs but because of their potency, especially in larger doses, they can knock out some of the normal reflex actions in which the sympathetic nervous system plays a critical role, specifically the effects of postural changes on the blood pressure.

If not for adequate sympathetic nervous system activity, when the human animal changes his posture from a lying or sitting position to a standing one, the blood volume would follow the laws of gravity and drop to the lower parts of the body. Blood pressure would drop precipitously with each change in posture unless there were some compensatory reflex. One of the roles of the sympathetic nervous system is to react immediately in this situation, narrowing the arteries and veins in the lower extremities to insure that blood does not pool in the legs. This prompt reflex maintains blood pressure at normal levels and protects us from fainting each time we change our posture.

Patients who are taking Guanethidine, and to a lesser extent Aldomet, may have a diminution in this reflex. If they stand up quickly they may suddenly feel dizzy or faint. This is called postural or orthostatic hypotension and is related to the antihypertensive action of the drug. These side effects are easily handled, however, if the patient remembers that he has a diminished reflex of this kind. He must remember to change his position slowly, sitting up in bed for a few minutes before rising, for example. If this is done slowly each time the position is changed, the reflexes reduced by the drug will have time to accommodate and the patient will protect himself from the possibility of fainting. Because of the postural effect of the drug, its antihypertensive effect can be enhanced by sleeping with the head slightly elevated, either on a few pillows or by placing several books under the legs of the headboard.

Recently, a new type of antisympathetic drug has become available for treatment of hypertension. Clonidine (Catapres®) affects the central nervous system to decrease the activity of the sympathetic nervous system. It is better tolerated by some patients than other of the sympatholytic drugs and has been a valuable addition to the management of hypertension.

Another effective class of antihypertensive drug, hydralazine (Apresoline®), and Prazosin (Minipress®), work directly as vasodilators or vascular relaxants. Taken orally, usually in conjunction with a diuretic, these drugs reduce the blood pressure directly by opening up the arteries and thereby decreasing the peripheral resistance. These drugs are interesting because they do not involve the sympathetic nervous system at all. They are effective taken orally, in several doses throughout the day, and hydralazine by injection can be given in an acute situation.

A combined drug which includes each of these classes of effective antihypertensive medication—reserpine, hydralazine, and the thiazide diuretics—is often used to manage high blood pressure. Physicians who are widely experienced in the management of hypertension may prefer to regulate the drugs separately, although the fixed combination is used by many.

A new class of drugs now being used in the management of hypertension is the beta-adrenergic blocking agents. Propanolol (Inderal®) is the only drug of this type available in the United States. They act by blocking the beta effects of the sympathetic nervous system, thus reducing the heart rate, decreasing the strength of the heart's contraction, and decreasing the cardiac output. As this occurs, the blood pressure is lowered. The beta-blockers are useful in the treatment of angina or other symptoms of ischemic coronary disease. They are also used to treat hypertension, especially when the blood pressure problem combines with severe arteriosclerotic heart disease to produce anginal pain. These drugs are especially valuable in the management of hypertension when the patient is also taking hydralazine because the beta-blockers prevent the increase in heart rate that may be a troublesome side effect of therapy with hydralazine.

Combined hydralazine and propanolol is useful to manage patients with severe hypertension who do not respond to other drugs or experience stubborn side effects with other therapies. Again the beta-blockers are usually given in combination with the oral diuretics on a varied dosage schedule. Although the adrenergic beta-blockers are not yet in frequent use for routine hypertension therapy, they can be a valuable addition to the known modes of treatment for hypertension. Recently it has also been shown that propanolol also decreases or blocks the production of renin by the kidney. This effect may be of importance in the treatment of patients with high blood renin levels or those who are refractory to other drugs.

There are two drugs that are used for the treatment of acute severe hypertension (hypertensive crisis) that must be given intravenously and only to closely monitored patients in the hospital. They are *nitroprusside,* a rapidly acting vessel dilator that is occasionally used in patients with acute heart attack who also have hypertension, and *Arfonad,* a drug that blocks neural transmission at the level of interneural connections. These drugs are not used for long-term management of hypertension.

SUMMARY

Most forms of hypertension, as I have noted, are not curable but must be treated with drugs and other forms of therapy throughout the patient's lifetime. Dr. Edward Freis, an eminent physician and researcher in the field, has suggested an approach similar to that used with diabetes. He emphasizes that the patient must be educated in a lifelong program of blood pressure control if he is to participate knowingly and willingly in an effective program of therapeutic regimens.

The information given in this chapter is directed toward that end; it goes somewhat beyond what is usually disseminated to the layman. While I think the material dispensed by busy physicians in their offices is fine, as far as it goes, I strongly believe the control of hypertension to be so vital that information usually given only to professionals has been included here. Too often have I heard physicians say in frustration, "If only my patients understood. . . ."

The material given in this chapter is vital—for your good health and your family's. Understood and acted upon, it suggests a magnificent opportunity for the significant control and prevention of cardiac, renal, and cerebrovascular disease.

Chapter 6

Cholesterol and Triglycerides: The Rational Reduction of High Lipid Levels

Cholesterol is the semidisreputable hanger-on of the coronary risk factor family. Because it is too subtle to appear openly as a complete outlaw, cholesterol has never actually been caught in the act of "causing" a heart attack. But, on the other hand, cholesterol has been at the scene of the crime far too often to be considered innocent of any part in its commission. So, although we do not have enough evidence to convict cholesterol as an arch "cause," we do know enough to suggest that rational adults approach the matter seriously.

The data indicting cholesterol are mainly circumstantial. This does not mean that the evidence is not strong, only that a definite causal relationship between human heart disease and cholesterol in the diet has not yet been conclusively demonstrated.

The major evidence indicting cholesterol is the finding on chemical analysis that cholesterol is the chief component of the atherosclerotic lesion that narrows and eventually occludes a coronary artery—the underlying cause of most heart attacks. Cholesterol is manufactured by the body, and the question of whether excess cholesterol in the diet causes deposition to atherosclerotic plaques is still unsettled. There is, however, a great deal of evidence that dietary intake of cholesterol plays a major role in the development of atherosclerosis.

Epidemiologic investigations (defined roughly as the study of large groups of people over long periods of time to determine which factors in a population are associated with which conditions) have demonstrated a striking relationship between dietary cholesterol and atherosclerosis throughout the world. In study after study, the cholesterol level in the blood has been found to have the strongest association with heart attacks and related cardiovascular disease. The higher the cholesterol level in an individual, the greater his risk of heart attack.

One of the best sources of epidemiologic information on the role of cholesterol in heart disease has been the famed Framingham study. Sponsored by the United States Public Health Service in a medium-sized, typical American city in central Massachusetts, this long-range program has followed participating members of the community for over twenty years. Periodic laboratory studies have been performed at regular intervals on this large group of people in order to gather complete health information. Meticulous records are kept by trained public health professionals; each illness and hospitalization is documented in an effort to obtain complete data on the lifelong health experience of more than 5,000 people sharing the same proximate environment.

When individual findings were correlated with outcome data in Framingham—that is, when the records of all the people who had suffered heart attacks were surveyed to see what they had in common—certain patterns emerged. One of the most significant findings of the Framingham study is that the risk of developing heart attacks seems to correlate directly with the level of cholesterol in the blood of participants. Furthermore, the data suggest a continuum of effect: people with low cholesterol levels have the lowest probability of developing heart attacks, while those with high cholesterol levels have a higher probability in what is considered to be a significant mathematical progression. The higher the cholesterol level, the more likely the chance of having a heart attack.

In a related analysis of the data, the Framingham group looked at triglyceride blood levels (another lipid normally found in the blood) and found that they are not as good a predictive factor as cholesterol. Further laboratory studies have suggested, however, that people who have a lipid abnormality that combines relatively or abnormally high cholesterol levels with abnormally high triglycerides may have a very high risk for the development of coronary artery disease.

In Sweden, a nine-year follow-up of more than three thousand men confirmed the Farmingham findings that high levels of plasma cholesterol were associated with increased risk of myocardial infarction. Men with high levels of blood lipids, both cholesterol and triglycerides, suffered the consequences of ischemic heart disease far more frequently than those who had low levels of both. This study also confirmed the belief that more than one risk factor adds to the likelihood of heart disease in more than just an additive fashion. When smoking was present in addition to elevated cholesterol, the risk of heart disease rose geometrically.

Normal Cholesterol Levels

In the United States, the normal cholesterol levels for adult males is generally set at 180 to 250 milligrams per 100 milliliters of blood, the American average being somewhere around 240 mg/100 ml. This concept of "normal" may be part of the problem, since at least one researcher in the field, Dr. Donald S. Frederickson, states that "individuals with cholesterol concentrations below 240 mg still have an increased risk of premature coronary disease."

He goes on to dispute another traditionally held belief concerning cholesterol levels. For years the "normal" levels of cholesterol have been stated in a range that increases with age. That is, the upper limit of normal for individuals twenty-nine years old and below is considered to be 240 milligrams per 100 milliliters of blood; for ages thirty to thirty-nine, the upper limit of normal is 270 mg/ml; for ages forty to forty-nine, the range has been up to 310 mg/ml; and for adults fifty years old and older, the upper limit of normal has beeen 330 milligrams. But Frederickson's recent work suggests that this increase in normal lipid levels with age is, in his words, not a "normal or healthy phenomenon." He challenges the belief that age should normally raise cholesterol levels and suggests that *all* adult Americans under the age of fifty-five whose cholesterol levels exceed 220 milligrams per 100 milliliters of blood should be considered for treatment of some kind. (Triglyceride levels, whose upper limits of normal have been considered to range from 140 mg/100 ml to 190, may deserve attention at 140 and above for all ages under fifty-five.)

Frederickson's beliefs are substantiated by heart disease findings in other parts of the world. In Japan, for instance, where the coronary disease rate until recent years has been quite low, doctors view cholesterol levels of 180 and above as conditions that warrant some concern. The generally high rate of heart disease in the United States suggests that our so-called normal levels reflect only the generally elevated levels of cholesterol throughout this country.

Many other epidemiologic studies have shown the same correlation between elevated cholesterol levels and heart attacks. Compelling evidence comes from statistics supplied by nations throughout the world which are codified by the World Health Organization and verified by respected medical groups in this country and elsewhere. In countries where diets are necessarily low in cholesterol—where proteins and fats of animal origin are scarce or costly—coronary heart disease is not prevalent. It is especially significant that as nations become wealthy—as their diets "improve" and become richer in costly foods such as red meat and dairy products—the incidence of coronary heart disease begins to rise. This has been the case in Japan, where the number of heart attacks has kept pace with the country's rising affluence, and in Israel, where "improved" diets appear to be reflected in rising coronary disease rates. In country after country, as the relatively cheap vegetable crop products are replaced with the more costly animal products that bespeak affluence, the risk of heart disease rises. Refined foods, meat and dairy products, and convenience foods are all part of the rich man's diet and all contribute to what has been called the American pattern of "environmental hyperlipidemia."

EARLY LABORATORY STUDIES

One of the first links in the chain of evidence connecting cholesterol to coronary artery disease and early death from heart attacks came from the unlikely laboratory of the Imperial Army of the Czar of All the Russias. Early in the 1900s a Russian army doctor named Ignatowsky spent most of his service, for reasons now lost in history, doing autopsies on the bodies of men who died while in the service of the czar. This was an extremely fortuitous situation, for it was almost impossible at that time to study the pathology of clogged arteries in a living human and postmortem examination has always been an excellent source of information of this kind.

Ignatowsky was perceptive and noticed that even in death there was a vast difference between the officers of the Imperial Army and the lowly foot soldiers. The common soldiers were men of peasant stock, very poor and possibly ill-fed, but they died with the remarkably clean, normal arteries of young men. In contrast, autopsies on officers who died at comparable ages revealed widespread atherosclerosis—the marked narrowing of many of the vital arteries, sometimes with the complete occlusion that was at that time thought only to occur in much older men. Interested, possibly bored with the life of an army doctor, and stimulated by this curious finding, Ignatowsky began to gather data to document the differences between the infantry men he autopsied who had no atherosclerosis and those officers of the same age who died with widespread clogging of the arteries.

One difference was immediately apparent. The officers were always well-nourished and frequently fat, while the foot soldiers were usually lean. The czar did not believe in feeding the peasants well, even when they were in his army. While the officers were supplied with meat and dairy products, the peasants of the infantry subsisted on black bread, perhaps some herring or other fish, and various grains and vegetables. They had almost no meat in their diets and little in the way of eggs or dairy products. In the ranks of the Russian army, there were few overweight foot soldiers.

In what has to be described as a creative leap of the research imagination, since no one had thought of it before, Ignatowsky postulated that it was their widely varying diets that caused the marked difference between the atherosclerosis-clogged arteries of the officers and the younger, healthier, "cleaner" arteries of the foot soldiers. In carrying this work further, Ignatowsky fortuitously chose to experiment by altering the diets of rabbits, one of the few species in which atherosclerosis can be produced by dietary manipulation alone.

Ignatowsky experimented by feeding rabbits the complete officers' diet of large amounts of eggs, butter, milk, meat, cakes, beer and sweets. The rabbits grew fat, and after observing them on this diet for a period of time, Ignatowsky sacrificed the animals and examined their arterial beds. In his fat rabbits he found widespread lesions similar to the atherosclerosis noted in the vessels of officers at autopsy. Through these and other related experiments, Ignatowsky concluded that it had to be something in the diet that effected the producton of atherosclerosis.

Some years later the relationship between cholesterol and atherosclerosis engaged the attention of another Russian doctor named Anitschkow. With slightly more background in biochemistry, he noted that the atherosclerotic plaques recovered post mortem in the early stages of their development contained cholesterol and various other fats. As these deposits matured they would calcify and harden, but at the early stages they were found to contain large amounts of cholesterol. Anitschkow repeated Ignatowsky's experiments with the rabbits, but instead of feeding them the officers' rich foods, he fed them cholesterol alone.

On this diet Anitschkow found that his rabbits soon developed high levels of cholesterol in their blood. When the animals were sacrificed and studied pathologically, this finding was correlated with extensive atherosclerotic narrowing of their blood vessels. Anitschkow postulated that the cholesterol carried by the blood was taken up by the inside layers of the vessels; as this cholesterol material built up and accumulated, the hard, clogging plaques of atherosclerosis were formed.

Ignatowsky's and Anitschkow's early work forms the basis for the dietary prevention of atherosclerosis. It is ironic that their findings were confirmed decades later by postmortem studies of the young, well-nourished American men who were killed during the Korean War. Physicians were stunned to find widespread and advanced atherosclerosis among these young and apparently healthy men. (Similar findings were later reported among the young men killed during the war in Vietnam.)

These discoveries radically altered attitudes in this country toward the causes of cardiovascular disease, because prior to this time atherosclerosis or "hardening of the arteries" was considered mainly a disease of the aged. Reports of the widespread prevalence of atherosclerosis among young men healthy enough to be drafted to fight a war suggested that this was a disease that was indeed epidemic, striking at all ages.

In other experimental work, atherosclerotic lesions have been produced by dietary manipulation in a variety of animals including monkeys, chickens, dogs, and guinea pigs. Most of these studies have required that diet be manipulated drastically and in some experimental animals hypothyroidism, achieved by inhibiting the activity of the thyroid gland, was required before atherosclerotic plaques developed. It is clear, however, that diets high in fats produce high lipid levels in the blood of the experimental animals studied, and when the arterial beds are examined widespread atherosclerosis is almost always present.

The work of Ignatowsky and Anitschkow showed that dietary cholesterol can play a primary role in the genesis of atherosclerosis. Along with data from Framingham and other epidemiologic studies showing that individuals with high blood levels of cholesterol have an increased incidence of heart disease, these findings indicate that it is eminently rational to suggest that the amount of cholesterol in the body be controlled by dietary and other means.

QUESTIONS OF CAUSE AND EFFECT

Again I must note that the causal role of high serum lipids—cholesterol and triglycerides—has not yet been completely demonstrated. In animals the evidence certainly suggests that it can be causal. Correlative evidence derived from human studies shows that people with high levels of cholesterol tend to have more coronary artery disease than those with low levels. Some have argued, however, that both of these conditions—high levels of cholesterol in the blood and high incidence of coronary artery disease—may be due to still a third abnormality not yet described, and thus high cholesterol levels may not be causally related to heart attacks.

Although the statistical evidence linking high cholesterol to heart disease is unmistakable, a number of questions yet remain. First, do high cholesterol levels in the blood cause the deposit of atherosclerotic plaques in the arteries or are both atherosclerosis and high serum cholesterol the result of something else, not yet identified, which predisposes to heart disease? Will reducing the cholesterol blood levels in people without coronary atherosclerosis prevent its development? In those who have already suffered a heart attack, will reducing cholesterol levels affect the chances of having still another attack? And, most important, will reducing cholesterol levels in the blood cleanse the arteries of existent atherosclerosis and in this way prevent heart attacks?

The important question of whether altering blood cholesterol will affect the development of atherosclerosis has been studied in a number of research sites; an important Finnish study of this question, conducted among patients living in two mental hospitals, required more than twelve years to complete. In one of the two hospitals the entire population was placed on a cholesterol-lowering diet for the first six years and the incidence of coronary heart disease was compared with that of the hospital which remained on its usual diet. During the second six-year period, the diets were reversed and the low cholesterol hospital reverted to a normal diet while the control hospital went on the low cholesterol regimen.

During the period of low cholesterol diet for each institution, the number of deaths from coronary heart disease was reduced considerably. (Total mortality from all causes was also lower but the authors caution that the numbers are too small to be statistically significant.) The extended period covered by this complex study allowed the researchers to make a fairly strong observation: "the change from the normal hospital diet to the cholesterol-lowering diet decreased the coronary heart disease death rate by about half, and the change from the cholesterol-lowering diet to the normal hospital diet more than doubled this death rate." (*Lancet*, Oct. 21, 1972, p. 838)

In the United States, at Mt. Sinai Hospital in New York, work begun by Dr. Norman Jolliffe in 1957 with members of the Anti-Coronary Club continues. Men who participate in this study adhere to the "Prudent Diet" designed around low-fat foods readily available in any supermarket. This long-term study has been effective in reducing cholesterol levels, especially in those subjects whose initial base-line levels are high—260 milligrams per 100 milliliters of blood. The men who adhere to this diet—and Mt. Sinai reports no lack of volunteers or enthusiasm among those who participate—have less than *half* the number of heart attacks experienced by men on the standard American diet.

This long-term experience with a free-living population is underscored by a study of men living at the Wadsworth Veterans Administration Hospital in California. The large number of men living there were randomly assigned to two different groups for meals. One group received the regular hospital diet while the other ate especially prepared low-fat meals. The results of this study, reported in 1969, suggested that modifying the cholesterol levels in adult men decreased their risk of heart attacks and indicated a causal relationship of some degree, since the group that ate the low-cholesterol, low-saturated fat diet had significantly fewer heart attacks. More work remains to be done in this study but its initial findings are extremely provocative.

In a recent animal study concerned with the reversibility of existing atherosclerosis, researchers at the University of Chicago and the University of Iowa placed a group of Rhesus monkeys on a high-cholesterol, high-saturated fat diet for eighteen months. At the end of this time all of the animals showed high cholesterol levels and those that died had severe and extensive atherosclerosis. The remaining animals were then divided into several groups, one continuing on the high-fat diet for another eighteen-month period while the others received a low-fat diet supplemented by polyunsaturated oil.

At the end of the second experimental period the monkeys on the high-fat diet again showed widespread atherosclerotic clogging of the arteries. But even more striking was the reduction in atherosclerosis noted in the monkeys on the low-fat diet. Cholesterol levels had fallen appreciably and significantly less atherosclerosis was found in the arteries of these animals. This study provided some hard evidence that a low-fat diet may cleanse the arteries of existing atherosclerosis. Monkeys, however, do not normally develop atherosclerosis on their usual diet, so the applicability of this study to humans remains in doubt.

Reversibility of coronary atherosclerosis in humans has not yet been demonstrated although there was a single report that atherosclerosis in the arteries of the legs was reversed by serum lipid manipulation in at least one type of lipid abnormality (Type V) and a recent report that very early atherosclerotic lesions may be reversible by manipulation of diet. Many physicians (myself included) have attempted to at least retard progression of atherosclerosis and possibly reverse the process in patients with severe disease who are very symptomatic and not surgical candidates by lowering cholesterol blood levels. The efficacy of this approach has yet to be proven.

In this country, the largest study of the prevention of recurrent heart attacks by drug treatment with cholesterol-lowering agents is the Coronary Drug Project, sponsored by the National Heart and Lung Institute and concluded 1975. Approximately ten thousand men with at least one documented myocardial infarction were randomly assigned to one of a number of drug regimens, and their clinical progress was followed for five years or more in over fifty cooperating clinics throughout the United States. The purpose of the project was to determine whether treatment to reduce cholesterol levels would decrease the incidence of subsequent heart attacks.

When all the data were examined at the completion of the Coronary Drug Project, it appeared that the modest reduction of blood cholesterol achieved with cholesterol-lowering drugs did not significantly alter the incidence of either mortality or recurrent myocardial infarction in this group of survivors of at least one heart attack. The lack of benefit as compared with previous studies may have been related to the fact that cholesterol was lowered only moderately by the drugs and the patients, all of whom had had at least one heart attack, may have had severe atherosclerosis prior to entering the study.

In broad outline this is the evidence on which we are asked to indict cholesterol: laboratory experiments that show that animals fed large amounts of cholesterol or cholesterol-containing foods develop atherosclerosis and narrowing of the arteries; the analysis of atherosclerotic plaques that show them to be composed mainly of concentrations of cholesterol; a few studies involving humans that show fewer heart attacks among groups fed low-cholesterol diets; and, most important, repeated strong epidemiologic evidence that shows a high degree of correlation between diets high in cholesterol and heart disease.

Although the case for altering dietary cholesterol is not yet absolutely conclusive, rational, thoughtful consideration of what we already know strongly suggests that Americans can and should reduce the amount of fat they ingest. Already there has been some sparse data to suggest that atherosclerosis already present in the human adult can be reduced by altering serum cholesterol levels. Modifying the diet of several free-living and institutionalized populations has indicated that the rate of coronary heart disease is reduced in those on low-fat diets, a finding that implies some benefit in preventing the development of atherosclerosis in children and young adults. So on these bases I recommend the value of low-cholesterol and low-saturated fat diets for everyone in an effort to control the spread of epidemic coronary artery disease and heart attacks.

THE "PRUDENT" DIET

The suggestions that follow are intended for symptom-free, healthy people. Those in whom physical examination or laboratory tests have disclosed some abnormality, or those with a strong family history of premature heart disease, should proceed even further and alter their diets considerably to achieve a more favorable lipid pattern. Suggestions for more vigorous dietary management begin on page 131.

For most people, however, some simple dietary changes, extremely easy and palatable to both the taste and the pocketbook, will effect some beneficial, long-term changes. Similar prudent measures have been endorsed by a number of health organizations, including the American Heart Association, the National Academy of Sciences—National Research Council, and the Council on Food and Nutrition of the American Medical Association.

Although it is wise for everyone to modify his diet and lower fat and cholesterol intake, in certain individuals such dietary changes are especially important. The first step in determining to what degree you must alter your diet is the sensible judgment of whether yours is a disease-prone family. Since the matter revolves about the prematurity of heart disease, a good test is at what age your parents or grandparents died and of what. If there are a distressing number of deaths under the age of fifty from heart disease in your family, you might consider your history suspect and further measures, including a visit to your physician and a laboratory determination of your body chemistry, are indicated.

If your family history is relatively free of early death from heart disease and if you are found to be in pretty good shape by your doctor, a rational plan of prudent eating should be instituted. If you are obese you will surely want to lose weight, and if you are diabetic you will want to keep your blood sugar levels within normal limits with the help of your physician and the diet and medication he prescribes for you.

For most families, the prudent diet requires only some awareness of the fat content of certain foods and a few judicious, often tasty, substitutions. Foods that are high in cholesterol and dietary fats are easily identified. As a rule of thumb, all animal fats and foods containing animal fats are high in saturated fats and therefore contain relatively large amounts of cholesterol. Saturated fats, which are known to be related to elevated blood levels of cholesterol and triglyceride are those which remain solid at room temperature, while the unsaturated fats which lower blood lipid levels are neither solidified nor hydrogenated and remain clear and liquid at room temperature. Butter, which is an animal product high in saturated fat, is solid or only softens at room temperature; corn oil, unless it is hydrogenated, remains liquid.

The source of most unsaturated cooking oils is vegetables—corn, soybean, safflower, sesame, and cottonseed—while saturated fats usually come from animal sources. The saturated fat in steak and other beef is white and solid at room temperature while unsaturated fish oil is liquid and usually clear enough to see through. Some nutritionists suggest that the polyunsaturated quality of vegetable cooking oils be preserved by refrigeration, and even then they remain liquid.

In this country, the main source of animal protein is beef and even lean beef contains a significant amount of saturated fat and cholesterol. Our prime beef has streaks of marbling throughout which are nothing more than fat within the meat that cannot be cut out. Without question, all of the visible fat on meats of any kind should be removed before cooking. Gravy made from meat drippings is full of fat and should be prepared well in advance of serving and then chilled so that all of the fat that solidifies on the surface can be skimmed off.

Other foods easily removed from a diet that seeks to reduce cholesterol intake are the organ or visceral meats. Liver, for instance, has a large amount of saturated fat and cholesterol in relation to its protein content; liver and its relatives, kidney, tripe, and sweetbreads, should be eaten infrequently. Various shellfish, although low in saturated fats, contain more of a substance similar to cholesterol than most other kinds of fish. Shrimp, crab, and lobster should be eaten less frequently than nonshell fish, although recently the prohibition on shellfish has been somewhat relaxed.

All dairy foods not specially prepared to reduce their fat content are high in cholesterol: whole milk, which contains large amounts of cholesterol and triglycerides, cheeses made with whole milk or cream, and cream in every form (sweet, iced, sour, half-and-half). Egg yolk is perhaps the most concentrated source of dietary cholesterol. People with known blood lipid abnormalities should adhere to a strictly egg-free diet and the cholesterol-free egg substitute now on the market should be used whenever possible. For all others moderation should rule. Except where clinically proven hypercholesterolemia exists, up to three eggs a week can be tolerated by most adults without significant elevations in cholesterol and triglyceride levels.

It should be emphasized that the egg you enjoy for a breakfast fairly low in calories is not the only source of egg yolk and its cholesterol in the diet. If you eat a substantial piece of cake you have probably taken in the better part of one egg. Most people are surprised by a glance through a pastry recipe book. Almost every cake or pastry recipe includes anywhere from one to six eggs and, since cooking, baking, or drying the egg yolk does not in any way change its cholesterol content, eggs ingested in this way still act to raise the lipid levels in the blood. Commercially prepared baked goods contain eggs and egg yolk in abundance; in fact, the more expensive the product, the more saturated fat it usually contains. Cakes and pastries are a source of cholesterol in the form of butter, too, since rich cakes contain large amounts of animal shortening and sometimes cream or milk as well.

One problem with the American diet revolves around its reliance on convenience-type prepared foods. Conditioned by a huge food industry that spends millions on advertising, American families increased their consumption of "store-bought" items many times over the past several decades. And it is a sad truth that many of these foods are extremely high in cholesterol.

Smoked and cured meats, for example—hot dogs, delicatessen meats, lunch meats, and cold cuts—are high in saturated fats (as well as in the salt that should be avoided by anyone with a tendency toward high blood pressure). The universal hamburger, whether purchased raw as ground meat or thoughtlessly consumed at a fast-food counter, is often composed of more than 30 percent fat. (Recent efforts to require the accurate labeling of ground meats should be supported by everyone.) Concerned housewives would do well to restrict their purchase of these foods and to raise their voices loud and clear to demand new federal limits on the amount of fat that is permitted by law in any of these prepared meat products.

The same is true of packaged cakes, snack foods, and baked goods. Usually prepared with saturated shortening and egg yolks (for "richness" and that much talked of "golden" color), almost all of the prepared cakes, cookies, and pies that you bring home from the store are high in fats as well as in "empty" refined sugar calories. If these products were required to be labeled, and if everyone understood the meaning of their contents, there is little doubt that the resulting lowered sales would lead to a rapidly improved product.

If the consumer were to demand it, and back up his demands with his pocketbook by refusing to buy such things as butter, cream, and other rich dairy products, there is no question that the American dairy industry would sponsor research that would result in tasty, improved, and healthful milk products significantly lower in saturated fats. When the sales figures underscore an informed shift to low-fat milk products, you can be certain that the industry's developmental efforts will be directed toward the improvement of these products.

The meat industry would also be responsive to a shift in the consumer dollar. There is no question that they can do much more to provide an economical source of protein significantly lower in saturated fats and cholesterol. There have already been a few reports of cattle bred to yield beef that is ten times higher in beneficial polyunsaturates. Since the ratio of polyunsaturates to saturates is effective in reducing the cholesterol levels in the blood, this beef was found to be useful in the dietary management of a group of healthy Australian subjects. Laboratory tests showed that within one month blood cholesterol levels among these subjects had dropped an average of 10 percent.

What to Eat

If you are aware of the foods which contain large amounts of saturated fat and cholesterol, you will find it relatively simple to reduce their intake significantly. There are a number of delicious and often less expensive foods that contain, for their weight and protein content, relatively low levels of the fats you want to avoid in order to lower cholesterol levels. Margarine, for example, is cheaper than butter. And almost all of these low-fat foods have the advantage of being lower in calories, a big plus for the vast numbers of people who want to lose even a few pounds.

In the main dish category concentrate on fowl, a wonderful food that is low in cholesterol, calories, and price. This means that chicken and turkey should be served at least twice a week; well-cooked, crisply drained duck can also be used on occasion. Young animals such as veal or spring lamb are relatively low in saturated fat, although again all visible fat should be removed before cooking. (Meats from young animals do not have the marbling seen in the meats of mature animals.)

Except for the mature cow, sheep, or pig, yielding beef, mutton, or pork, other meats are relatively low in cholesterol if all visible fat is removed before cooking or allowed to drain off into the broiler.

Pork products are especially high in cholesterol and should be avoided whenever possible. A sensible diet, low in calories and cholesterol, should thus revolve around fish and fowl, veal, lamb and very lean beef on occasion.

A diet that strives to reduce cholesterol intake should feature fish two to four times a week. All kinds of "finny" fish are quite low in saturated fats and cholesterol and contain primarily unsaturated fats that help in reducing lipid levels. All shellfish are high in a substance that is like cholesterol, so shrimp, crab, and lobster should be eaten no more than once a week. Fish can be prepared in a number of ingenious ways, although the prudent cook would eliminate butter in preparation. Try corn oil margarine instead, or cook the fish in a seasoned sauce made with tomato juice and onions, green pepper, and celery. Try eating filets of the larger fish if you are a lifelong beefeater. Broiled, with lemon juice and seasoning or a glaze of olive oil, thick fish filets provide few calories, little cholesterol, and a lot of eating satisfaction. If you eat in restaurants frequently, be sure to specify that no butter be used in preparing your fish.

Canned fish, such as salmon, tuna and sardines, are low in saturated fats. Even those packed in oil are low in saturates and can be eaten as desired. If calorie control is also a goal, those fish packed in water or broth are preferred, whereas those in oil should be well drained before eating. Sardines, salmon, and tuna should be used extensively at lunch, either alone or in salads. The semi-delicacies of the fish family, herrings pickled or packed in oil or cream sauce, are also low in cholesterol when compared to the amount of protein and satisfaction they provide, and they can also be eaten on occasion.

Substituting fowl and fish of various sorts for beef can become a lifelong eating habit that is quite rewarding as far as the palate and the blood lipid levels are concerned. Although our society appears to be built around steak and roast beef, this is no more than a convenient—and expensive—cultural trait. At a time when nutritionists and cardiologists express alarm at the almost 45 percent fat content of the American diet, it should be pointed out that this pattern is not a necessity and that food habits can and should be changed. Having lean, well-trimmed beef only once a week, or ordering filet of whitefish or broiled Dover sole instead of steak in a restaurant, can also become a habit and a healthful source of a great deal of dietary satisfaction.

Among the dairy products, whole milk and whole milk cheeses should be avoided. Cottage cheese, pot cheese, and farmer cheese are made from the curds of milk and tend to be lower in fats. Among the hard cheeses, try to select those that are made of skim milk. Yogurt is marvelous, especially in the new flavored varieties; most are formulated to contain little saturated fat. Yogurt is also useful as a topping for fruit, sweetened with a little sugar or honey, or in place of mayonnaise to bind together tuna or salmon into a tasty luncheon salad.

In place of butter, which need never be eaten, there are excellent margarines made of corn oil and other oils that are high in polyunsaturates and low in saturated fats. The soft margarines that come in small tubs are especially useful because oils must be hydrogenated or hardened to some extent to produce stick margarines. This increases the level of saturated fat and, although not adding to the cholesterol content, to some degree it negates the benefits of replacing butter with margarine. The soft margarines remain low in cholesterol and higher in polyunsaturates and should be chosen over the harder stick variety whenever possible.

It is also a good idea to always read the label, remembering that the ingredient listed first predominates. You will want to select margarines whose list of ingredients begins with liquid oil, usually corn, soybean, safflower, or cottonseed. Cooking oils should be chosen in the same way and refrigerated to preserve their polyunsaturated qualities.

Cream and half-and-half should be avoided. Try lightening your coffee with skim milk or, if this is not adequate, use whole milk. The taste is almost the same and you will probably be much better off than if you chose the dry powdered "creamers." Unless reformulated by the time this appears in print, most of the powdered coffee whiteners are based on coconut oil, an extremely concentrated source of saturated fat. Avoid these even though the label may read something like "vegetable oil solids." In its present form, even a teaspoonful of this stuff in several cups of coffee can greatly increase the daily intake of saturated fat.

Fruits, very low in cholesterol and saturated fat, can be eaten without exception and almost all vegetables can be enjoyed without limit. Most nuts are high in saturated fats and should be avoided, although some walnuts, pecans, and almonds are permitted on occasion. Most breads and grain products contain little in the way of saturated fat and cholesterol, although some of the expensive white breads and fancy rolls may contain eggs. Again read the label since most products of this kind are required to be carefully described.

Furthermore, most commercially prepared products boast about their egg content either in their advertising or on the label so it is usually easy to determine which product to avoid. Coconut and chocolate are extremely high in calories and high in saturated fat and should be avoided. When it comes to candy and packaged bakery products, in general the less you spend the less saturated fat you will buy, since most of the ingredients that contain cholesterol, like butter and eggs, are expensive and tend to raise the price of the product.

If obesity is not a problem, soft drinks are permitted in

limited amounts since they contain no saturated fats. They are high in sugar and relatively "empty" calories, however, and should be taken in only moderate quantities. Do not add ice cream if you are trying to keep your weight down and your cholesterol levels low. Alcohol and mixed drinks, again if they contain no milk or cream, are also relatively low in saturated fats and may be taken in moderation. Remember, though, alcohol is extremely high in calories and contributes mightily to any weight problem you may be trying to solve. Large amounts of alcohol, taken on a steady basis, are extremely deleterious to the health for a wide variety of reasons. In addition to their destructive action on the liver, they also raise the lipid levels of the blood. Chronic alcoholics frequently have high lipid levels secondary to the ingestion of large amounts of alcohol carbohydrate and to the subsequent damage of the liver.

Although coffee and tea are all right as far as cholesterol is concerned, it is again best to drink these stimulants only in moderation. (The peculiar role of heavy coffee drinking in the development of heart attacks is discussed further on page 276.) The use of cream should be avoided, but sugar, except in certain types of severe hyperlipidemia and in patients with diabetes, can be used in moderation.

Among other miscellaneous foodstuffs not permitted on a low cholesterol diet are avocados, bacon, cream cheese, potato chips, popcorn, and olives.

SUGGESTED DAILY MENUS

A typical daily menu for a family concerned with its intake of saturated fats and cholesterol would begin with the usual breakfast of fruit or juice, followed by a dish of hot or cold cereal with skim milk and fruit if desired. Corn oil margarine can be used as desired and, except where weight loss is also a goal, one or two slices of toast may be enjoyed.

Various forms of fish may also be eaten in the morning, as is the custom in England and the Scandinavian countries. An egg should be eaten no more than three times a week, and bacon, sausage, and other pork products should be avoided. Coffee, tea, or another breakfast beverage completes the meal.

For lunch and dinner, salads and various vegetables without butter can be eaten as desired. Salads can be prepared with vinegar or lemon juice and a polyunsaturated oil. Mayonnaise, a combination of egg yolk and oil, should be omitted or used sparingly. Since egg yolk is the most concentrated form of cholesterol, it should be avoided in any form such as salad dressings or commercially prepared baked goods. Fat-free broths or soups that have been prepared from permitted foods are allowed, although commercially canned soups and cream soups of any kind are usually high in cholesterol and saturated fats. Sandwiches made with margarine on the bread and tuna, salmon, sardine, or peanut butter filling can be used for convenience if you are not counting calories.

The meats that compose the main meal should be primarily veal or young lamb; the meat should be trimmed of visible fat and broiled whenever possible. Fowl of any type and fish can be eaten as desired, although care should be taken that no butter is used in the preparation.

How to Cheat

A word here on moderation. Since I personally rate cities on the quality of their ice cream and the number of interesting flavors available, I cannot in good conscience prescribe that the reader never again enjoy the special delight of a dish of ice cream. On the other hand, I must warn that ice cream, like so many other delightful things in life, is full of saturated fat and cholesterol. (Those who have clinically established elevated cholesterol levels need read no further; they really should *never* indulge in high cholesterol cheating.)

I have resolved the problem by a judicious degree of immoderate moderation. When absolutely nothing else will do, I enjoy a dish of ice cream. In order to avoid hating myself, however, I do this infrequently—certainly no more often than two or three times a month—and I limit my indulgence to a single dip of really great ice cream. (Ice cream freaks, of which I am one, know that a spoonful of a really distinguished product is far superior to a large amount of inferior glop.)

The same thing must be said, of course, about other elements of what you perceive as the good life. If there are no clinical contraindications, and if your family history does not suggest that cholesterol levels might be a source of concern, then you might develop your own way of handling an occasional high cholesterol treat. If a good steak is absolutely basic to your enjoyment of living, by all means have one—infrequently, rather than regularly, and preferably on a day when you have not also chosen to enjoy an egg for breakfast.

The same attitude should prevail in our thinking about childrens' diets. We just do not know enough about the long-term effects of a drastically altered diet to recommend that all children be strictly limited in cholesterol intake. Eggs, milk, and red meat are probably necessary for their proper growth, but again moderation must be the key. If there is a family history of lipid abnormality (elevated triglycerides or cholesterol), diabetes, gout, or heart disease, it is probably a good idea to check the child as early as possible. In a fascinating study of infants born to mothers with known hyperlipidemias, blood was taken from the umbilical cord at birth and tested in the delivery room for cholesterol. Results indicated that babies at high risk could be identified at birth and that it is reasonable to assume that dietary modification begun early in life could substantially affect the later expression of familial hypercholesterolemia.

For children from relatively disease-free families the indications are not so clear-cut. We do know that obesity is a difficult condition that starts early in life. If your chubby two-year-old shows signs of growing into a fat three-year-old, you might talk to your pediatrician about substituting skim milk for whole and cutting down a bit on red meat and eggs. Since dietary habits begun in childhood stay with us for good or ill throughout our lives, it is probably a good idea to avoid the empty calories of snack foods that are high in sugar and starch and low in practically everything else, including flavor. Fill the refrigerator with fruit and vegetable snacks; the kids will look better, live longer, and have fewer dental cavities in the bargain. Forget the old saw that the fat babies are the cute and healthy ones and direct your efforts to a sensible, well-balanced diet that is low in fats and sugar.

Moreover, since motherhood is reputedly the most potent force on earth, try harnessing this power to get more nutrition in the foods you buy. Again the real power lies in your purse; the junk that does not sell motivates the industry to develop something that will. Write letters, raise your voice for more nutrition, fewer calories, and far less sugar and fat.

FURTHER RESTRICTED DIET

People who are at some risk for elevated cholesterol should begin by identifying themselves. Since it is not yet feasible to screen everybody between the ages of twenty-five and fifty-nine, knowledgeable individuals with any of the following in their background should be checked for lipid levels: family history of premature death from heart disease or stroke, parental history of vascular or heart disease appearing before the age of fifty, hypertension, obesity, diabetes, gout or elevated uric acid levels. Postmenopausal women and those with liver problems or low thyroid levels should be under doctor's care since they also can have lipid abnormalities.

Any of these findings should signal the prudent individual to consult his physician since cholesterol levels can be managed by a comfortable continuum of methods. First the doctor recommends weight loss for those who are too heavy or frankly obese. Decreasing the weight significantly decreases lipid levels. During the period of active loss both cholesterol and triglycerides go down markedly even in patients with relatively advanced abnormalities. When the patient reaches his ideal body weight and resumes his regular diet where weight is no longer being actively lost, the lipid levels may continue at the lower rate, or in certain individuals may rise again. If cholesterol and triglycerides remain elevated while normal body weight is maintained, the physician may elect to use one of the other methods of lowering blood lipid levels.

(In the same way that weight loss reduces blood lipids, dietary management of diabetic patients will also reduce serum lipids, in most patients. The recommended diet is low in carbohydrates, and is used under the strict supervision of the physician in conjunction with antidiabetic medications.)

Apart from weight reduction, diet is the keystone of therapy for all elevated blood lipids. In a recent issue of *Modern Concepts of Cardiovascular Disease,* a publication of the American Heart Association, Dr. Donald S. Frederickson makes a provocative statement: "Exactly how most dietary maneuvers lower lipoprotein levels is not known, but *they are effective.* Often no other treatment is required. . . ."

Your physician will probably want to check your cholesterol and triglyceride levels at monthly intervals as the dietary regimen continues. This is a good way of checking on adherence to the special diet and the patient should take this opportunity to ask questions and request specific information.

Dr. Frederickson suggests that diet alone be tried for at least eight weeks, or a minimum of two patient visits, to clear up any misconceptions concerning the regimen to be followed. If after this period cholesterol and triglyceride levels remain elevated, most consultants agree that drug treatment should be instituted. The exact point at which drug therapy should be begun depends on the physician's evaluation of the individual's problem, but somewhere around 300 mg/100 ml is the usual cutoff figure.

LIPOPROTEIN PHENOTYPING

Like so many of the medical problems of the past, elevated blood lipids have recently been the subject of intensive scrutiny with new improved materials and laboratory techniques. As a result of remarkable work, much of it done under Dr. Frederickson's aegis at the National Heart and Lung Institute, people with proven lipid abnormalities can avail themselves of these advances in the typing of hyperlipidemias. Called *phenotyping,* this laboratory blood study identifies the pathway of the abnormal lipoprotein transport and allows the doctor to prescribe a drug and diet regimen that is specifically tailored to this type of abnormality.

Using a process called electrophoresis that involves no more than a blood sample and a good laboratory, this technique separates the lipoproteins into characteristic bands. The patterns of the bands on electrophoresis correlated with the levels of cholesterol and triglycerides in the blood have defined five major types of hyperlipidemia and a number of types that may be variants or combinations of the major types. Since each is amenable to a specific form of treatment, phenotyping is important in the investigation of those cases that do not respond to general diet therapy.

Electrophoretic phenotyping also suggests certain familial patterns. Genetics appears to play a role in certain types of elevated blood lipids, and the physician may recommend a study of other family members when phenotyping discloses specific abnormalities. Its actual role is not entirely clear, but inheritance appears to determine the individual's type or category of abnormality while his choice of food, and possibly his level of activity, determines the actual level.

In order to determine the specific abnormality of the lipo-protein pattern, your physician will draw a small sample of blood. Since we want to know about underlying conditions rather than about the fat content of your most recent meal, this is usually a fasting blood specimen, drawn from your arm in the morning before any food is eaten that can affect the pattern. Your physician will also give specific instructions about discontinuing certain other drugs for a period of time before the sample is drawn in order to avoid any unintentional contamination. The test for lipoprotein phenotyping is not done immediately after a coronary episode or heart attack because these events can also produce a specious finding.

The lipoproteins are described in Chapter 4. In general they are the carriers of the fat molecules in the blood serum; the patterns they make reflect any abnormality of the transport system, and allow the doctor to make inferences about the type of hyper-lipidemia that may be present. Once the phenotype is known the physician can prescribe a drug and diet regimen that is specific to the needs of the patient—and often to his family as well since several kinds of abnormalities may also appear in blood-related individuals.

DIETARY AND DRUG TREATMENT FOR
SPECIFIC TYPES OF HYPERLIPIDEMIAS

Most patients with elevated lipid levels prove to have hyper-lipoproteinemia that is identified as Type 2A, 2B, 3, or 4. Type 2A is characterized by high cholesterol levels with normal triglycer-ides, Type 4 shows normal or slightly elevated cholesterol and high triglycerides, whereas Types 2B and 3 have elevations of both cholesterol and triglycerides. In their mild form, which is the usual case, all of these types respond well to a program of weight control and prudent diet. The rare, severe form of Type 2A, characterized by high cholesterol levels (over 500), requires stringent reduction of the amount of saturated fat in the diet along with conscientious elimination of all foods containing cholesterol. Such strict dietary changes usually effect a significant drop in the abnormal cholesterol levels, although other measures, including drugs and rarely even surgery, may be necessary.

Type 4, with its characteristic elevated triglyceride levels, is often helped dramatically by diets that are low in carbohydrates. When alcohol is restricted or eliminated altogether and calories reduced by limiting carbohydrates, the weight drops and there is usually an appreciable decrease in the triglyceride level of the blood and normalization of the lipid patterns.

Type 2B, also known as combined hyperlipidemia or CHL, characterized by elevations of both cholesterol and triglycerides, is frequently associated with high uric acid, gout, obesity, and diabetes. It is quite common and has a high correlation with coronary disease. Weight loss and decreased dietary cholesterol intake are frequently effective in correcting this abnormality.

The relatively rare Type 3 is also characterized by moderate elevations of both cholesterol and triglycerides. It has a different electrophoretic pattern from Type 2B, however, and usually responds to drug and diet therapy. Type 3 is less common than Types 2 and 4 and is a familial trait.

Types 1 and 5 are seen far less frequently and are often accompanied by other systemic disorders. Type 1 is a rare inherited form of hyperlipidemia seen mostly in children under the age of ten who also have a severe intolerance to fat. They may have characteristic abdominal pain and suffer attacks of pancreatitis. Type 5 is characterized by very high levels of triglycerides along with elevated cholesterol. Patients found to fall into these two rarely seen types must have a special diet that is specifically designed to cope with these abnormalities.

Specific dietary information for each of the types of elevated lipids is available from your local heart association. If your abnormality is severe, your physician will probably recommend that you secure a diet book that describes specific menus in detail. You will find his experience and suggestions invaluable to a long-term dietary control of hyperlipidemia, and I urge you to establish a relationship that allows for consideration and consultation on both sides.

DRUG TREATMENT OF HIGH CHOLESTEROL LEVELS

When diet does not succeed in lowering cholesterol and triglyceride levels below the 300 mg mark, most physicians consider the use of a drug adjunct. The drugs available today are effective, easy to take, and specially formulated for use in certain types of hyperlipidemias.

Dextro- or D-thyroxine was developed after it was noted that people with hyperthyroidism—overactivity of the thyroid gland leading to increased production of the thyroid hormone—appeared to have lowered cholesterol levels in the blood. Conversely, patients with hypothyroidism or decreased levels of thyroid hormone usually have abnormally elevated cholesterol.

The thyroid hormone itself is not used because it has many other effects, including acceleration of the heart rate, excessive nervousness, sweating, and weight loss. (In its pure form, used as an adjunct to weight loss, it causes considerable stress to the cardiovascular system and poses some risk.) Dextro-thyroxine was formulated to retain the cholesterol-lowering effect without accelerating the body metabolism or causing other side effects. It successfully lowers cholesterol in Types 2 and 3, but does retain some of the effects of the pure thyroid hormone and produces side effects similar to hyperthyroidism in some patients. Since these may include arrhythmias or extra beats that can be hazardous in people with underlying heart disease, dextro-thyroxine must be used under the careful supervision of a physician.

Dextro-thyroxine was one of the cholesterol-lowering medications used by the Coronary Drug Project in its nationwide study of men who have had heart attacks. This carefully monitored research program noted no significant decrease in the incidence of heart attacks or sudden death among men on this drug. When a number of men on dextro-thyroxine showed electrocardiographic evidence of ventricular arrhythmias, the drug was discontinued and it is no longer recommended for patients with a history of heart disease.

In otherwise normal individuals, however, dextro-thyroxine is an effective drug and is used by physicians to lower cholesterol levels in certain selected persons.

Another drug used to reduce cholesterol levels developed from the finding that premenopausal women have a lower cholesterol level than men. Women who menstruate also have less coronary artery disease and a markedly reduced tendency to develop myocardial infarction or sudden death. Since the presence of estrogens differentiates premenopausal women from all others, estrogens were also included in the original design of the Coronary Drug Project. Although estrogens had previously been shown to lower cholesterol and decrease the incidence of heart attacks, they were dropped from the Coronary Drug Project, both in low and high doses, because they appeared to carry an increased risk for the development of thromboembolic phenomena, or blood clots. There was also no evidence that estrogen therapy in men produced any significant lowering in the rate of heart attacks or in the incidence of sudden death. Its side effects of breast enlargement, loss of libido, and feminization were not outweighed by any marked beneficial effects so estrogenic therapy for the purpose of improving the outlook for heart disease in men at some risk is not widely prescribed at this time.

Nicotinic acid, the B-vitamin niacin, is an effective cholesterol-lowering agent. It is the drug of choice for treatment of Type 5 hypercholesterolemia and is effective in other types as well. The drug does have some bothersome side effects but is well tolerated by most of the patients who are treated with it. Although it may produce signs of vasodilatation—throbbing headaches, flushing, or pounding in the head shortly after taking the drug—nicotinic acid is effective and is used by many physicians to lower cholesterol levels in patients who are able to tolerate its effects. Data from the Coronary Drug Project suggest it does not decrease the incidence of heart attacks in patients who have already had at least one heart attack.

A relatively new drug, available only in the last ten years or so, is called clofibrate (Atromid S®). This is an effective pharmacologic agent that lowers the plasma triglycerides and cholesterol levels by 10 to 15 percent.

Atromid, which was also studied in the Coronary Drug Project, is the drug of choice to treat Types 3, 4, and 5. Although there were reports of occasional extra beats or gastrointestinal disturbances, clofibrate was used by most people without discomfort or side effects of any kind.

Atromid has also proved an interesting drug in several other respects. In three large studies, two in England and one in the United States, it was observed that whether plasma lipids were lowered or not, people on the drug appeared to have fewer heart attacks and fewer episodes of sudden death. The reason for these startling findings is not clear although research efforts continue. It may be some subtle effect on the lipids that is not measured by the usual blood tests, or it may be something quite apart from its known cholesterol-lowering effects. Clofibrate may affect blood clotting mechanisms by altering the propensity for blood platelets to aggregate and for this reason may be effective in preventing heart attacks.

I emphasize that this is still highly questionable material, extremely inconclusive, and under intense research scrutiny all over the world. It is interesting that the Coronary Drug Project did not corroborate or confirm the beneficial effects seen in earlier studies.

A new class of drugs, only recently available, are the resins, Cholestipol® and Questran® being the only two available at the time of publication. Different from other cholesterol-lowering agents, resins go through the gastrointestinal tract but are not absorbed from the gut into the body. As they pass through the intestines they pull out the cholesterol that is available. The resins do this through their ability to absorb the bile salts, which are formed in the liver and are secreted into the gut with the bile. The bile salts contain large quantities of cholesterol and are the principal means by which cholesterol is excreted. They aid in the digestion of fats and ordinarily are reabsorbed and used over and over.

When the resins attach to the bile salts, however, they prevent their reabsorption by the gut and force them to be excreted. The liver must then form new bile salts, forcing the excretion of more cholesterol from which the salts are formed.

The resins are quite effective in lowering cholesterol levels, but they are difficult to take and poorly tolerated by many patients. In some patients the loss of a significant amount of the bile salts and the poor absorption of fat causes a bloated and gassy feeling, and some few individuals may develop constipation. The resins are usually taken with a large amount of liquid and their sandy consistency is sometimes successfully disguised in fruit juice. A mild laxative and some vitamins are sometimes added to the regimen.

The resins are effective drugs and are extremely useful in patients with classic Type 2A, which is characterized by high levels of cholesterol. In patients with flagrant hypercholesterolemia, the resins are quite necessary and their side effects must be overcome;

in some patients with lesser forms of elevated lipids they are also used with benefit.

SURGICAL TREATMENT OF HYPERCHOLESTEROLEMIA

The most extreme form of treatment for elevated cholesterol, used only in patients in whom a flagrant Type 2A condition produces consistently high blood levels, is surgery. In patients with a strong family history of heart attacks in both males and females at very early ages, it is sometimes necessary to reduce these dangerously high levels of lipids by an ileal bypass operation. This method of removing the ileum or short-circuiting the bowel reduces the amount of intestinal area that is available for reabsorption of bile salts and the cholesterol they contain.

Surgery is a drastic form of therapy for hypercholesterolemia and is used only in those patients whose high levels of blood cholesterol place them at high risk for heart attacks. Surgery of this kind is not done at every hospital and is considered only when nothing else is effective.

Chapter 7

Stress and How to Live With It: The Coronary-Prone Personality

Since everyone is exposed to considerable stress—sometimes chronic and sometimes acute—in the course of a normal lifetime, it is helpful to have a good working definition. According to Webster, stress is "a physical, chemical, or emotional factor (as trauma, histamine, or fear) to which an individual *fails* to make a satisfactory adaptation and which causes physiologic tensions that may be a contributory cause of disease."

The operant words here are the negative: "*fails* to make a satisfactory adaptation." Wise men have always known that the way we interact with our environment determines the amount of stress we suffer. The things that happen to us are important, of course, but our response to them and to our environment determines their effect on us. A number of people exposed to the same difficult situation respond in a variety of ways and this continual pattern of response determines—and is determined by—the individual personality. People who respond calmly to stress are considered to have a stoic personality, while people who react emotionally and volatilely are usually called high strung, or worse.

In the last twenty years or so, numerous medical investigations have demonstrated a definite correlation between stress and coronary heart disease. This relationship between emotional stress and atherosclerotic heart disease has been studied extensively in an effort to learn what can be done to identify and help those people who appear to possess the classic coronary-prone personality. Prospective studies, retrospective studies, chemical analyses, and psychosocial surveys have all been undertaken in an effort to determine why certain people develop heart disease while others, often with the same or worse physical background, do not.

Stress manifests itself in other physiological ways. Ulcers, colitis, asthma, and certain allergies have all been related in some patients to the effects of prolonged stress. But the heart appears to act as its major target and to occupy the central role. This relationship is not new: old-fashioned novels speak of people who are lionhearted or fainthearted, heartsick, or heartbroken. In modern literature, in the age of anxiety, people die of disappointment, of frustration over failing to achieve their goals, or over desires not fulfilled; in more dramatic terms people are portrayed as dying of fear or of sudden emotional upset.

Although in many instances these are fictional situations for heightened dramatic impact, good writers always accurately reflect reality in addition to the temper of their times. The fact is that instances of death or heart attack or other disease states following emotional upset or as the capstone of a stressful life are well documented in the medical literature.

THE OMNIPRESENCE OF STRESS

Folk wisdom holds that only the dead are free of problems, and there are few people alive today who would quarrel with that. Stress is quite literally everywhere, and always has been, but modern man, struggling to stay afloat in a hostile sea, appears to have a particular nemesis in the strains of twentieth-century living. For modern man, quite unlike his forebears, can do little when he encounters stress in his life. Although he is endowed biologically with the same responses (the sympathetic nervous system activates the adrenal glands to prepare the body to fight or flee, just as it did when prehistoric man came upon a sabre-toothed tiger), when modern man senses danger in the form of his boss, heavy traffic, or the Internal Revenue Service, he can usually only fret, or fume, or explode—or have a heart attack. It is this inability to discharge the hastily summoned energy that causes man such great difficulty in handling today's stress.

In the genuinely threatening situation involving physical danger, man's survival depended on the increased blood flow and rapidly stepped up blood pressure provided by a highly responsive sympathetic nervous system. In modern life, especially among those people who habitually overreact to stress, these reserves are called up almost daily; every difficult situation is perceived as a major threat and the body is taxed to provide added powers that may never be used.

The man who blows his top at a delay on the telephone is responding inappropriately with a large outpouring of the chemical mediators known as sympatetic catecholamines. His sympathetic nervous system is activated and the heart immediately begins to work harder. His blood pressure rises, blood flow is increased, and his body is prepared to grapple with a tiger—and all twentieth-century man can do is shout at the operator, or, even more frustrating, talk back to a recording.

This destructive pattern is easily recognized in some people. Everyone has to let off steam once in a while, and an occasional noisy release of frustration may be good for the human animal. In other people the pattern is less overt; the same emotional response produces little in the way of outward display. Constant reactions of this kind, whether apparent or controlled and hidden, are wearing to the organism, however, and people who overreact to relatively "normal" stress by calling up their reserves may eventually have to pay for these inappropriate responses with physical illness.

It is easy to tell a patient to slow down, to relax, and to stop worrying. It is also fairly simple to counsel a patient to stop reacting to every crisis in his life as though it were of life-threatening importance: a missed traffic light, a son with a beard, or a business deal that falls through are simply not of the same magnitude as the sabre-toothed tiger that stalked primitive man and should not stimulate the same outpouring of emotion and catecholamines as that damned tiger.

Moderation with regard to emotions can be achieved but it is not easy. One way is to consider that there is a kind of spectrum of emotional response, a standard developed by each individual and against which he can measure the appropriateness of his responses. For example, if the most serious genuinely life-threatening stress is to be handled with the maximum response, a missed telephone call should clearly rate only a small fraction of the maximum reaction. Kids with long hair and short manners and other fairly constant irritations should rate no more than a flicker on the scale of emotion.

A serious family situation, natural disaster, war, or loss of income all deserve and require the maximum response. The healthy body is ingeniously equipped to supply the extra energy that you need to cope with these serious, very real threats. But a fight with your wife (usually over the kid's long hair), or a boss who expects too much and pays too little, or a car that fails to start on cold mornings—depending on the circumstances—probably requires no more than a moderate physiological response. And all the other minor stresses of modern life should be handled with as small an emotional investment as is possible.

The point is, of course, to gain some insight into the way we react to the stress of living. If you give everything the maximum response, then clearly you are burning your emotional reserves at too rapid a rate. There is no question that living today is fraught with peril, just as it was when the sabre-toothed tiger roamed the earth. But a great deal of the stress that we respond to today is the kind that is of little importance in the long run and about which we can do absolutely nothing. These include traffic jams, the weather, the stock market, the economy, world politics, national politics to a large extent, an evening that turns out to be a waste of time, or an appointment that is canceled at the last minute—among many others. Remember, no matter how you rant and rave on the platform, the train that is delayed almost every morning will come no sooner.

To save wear and tear on your system, and to avoid the continual responses that lead to a wide variety of systemic illnesses, you must decide for yourself how and when you will respond maximally to specific stress. A good way to start is to develop the ability to determine which of the many stresses you are exposed to are entirely beyond your control and which must be dealt with by an active response.

Some people find that they gain perspective on the importance of their problems by talking them over with someone else. A good friend or mate whose patience and counsel are a source of insight and control can often fill this role. Sometimes just verbalizing the problem, "talking it out" to someone else, helps you to properly evaluate its importance. If there is no one with whom you are able to establish this kind of association, your family doctor or clergyman can be helpful as a sympathetic listener. Occasionally, if your problems are really overwhelming, a short session with a psychiatrist may be of value. Everyone, however, needs his own still small voice, functioning within, tirelessly repeating the words of ultimate wisdom: *Never worry about things over which you have no control.*

Simple words, really, but I am persuaded that mental and physical well-being can be sought through their wisdom. Each individual must use the insight he possesses to distinguish those situations over which he has some control from those in which he has little or none. And in today's world, most daily frustration falls into the latter category.

There is no point in discussing stress unless we can also give some insight as to how to avoid dying of its effects. While there is no "vaccine" or "miracle drug" available for the control of stress, there are ways to learn to live in spite of it. For those who are concerned with their own personal risk of heart attack, this chapter is organized in the following way.

First, there is a discussion of what happens to the human body under stress—the physiology of stress. Next, there is a brief overview of the many things outside the body that are known to produce stress: the job, one's marital status, where you live, how you live, and so on. Advice then follows on how to survive mourning or the less serious but still formidable stress of business or financial reverses, two strains closely associated with the occurrence of sudden death or premature disease. Last, there is a review of the important research that has opened up the field of stress-related illness and sudden death, especially as it relates to the concept of the coronary-prone personality.

The Physiology of Stress

In an effort to identify and aid those people whose reaction to stress may lead them to a heart attack, researchers have carefully studied the effect of stress on the living organism. Ingenious experiments involving animals in the laboratory and humans in both free-living and institutionalized populations have sought to describe exactly what takes place in the body when a living system is subjected to stress.

Many of the observed effects of stress have had to do with the activity of the sympathetic nervous system. As noted in the discussion of the role of the cardiovascular system in the maintenance of life, the sympathetic nervous system is the emergency system that comes into play when the organism is threatened. It is classically described as the system that prepared the individual for fight or flight.

A beautifully responsive system, absolutely essential to the life of man in his environment, the sympathetic nervous system acts through its chemical mediators, adrenalin and noradrenalin (also called epinephrine and norepinephrine, respectively), which are released from sympathetic nerve endings and from the adrenal glands. The action of this system causes an immediate cascade of physiologic effects that are needed to help the threatened organism to protect itself—or to run to preserve its life.

Adrenalin causes the heart to beat more strongly and rapidly, thus increasing the amount of blood flow to the body. This stronger, more rapid contraction of the heart increases the cardiac output of blood at once. It also redistributes the blood, sending increased supplies to those areas likely to need it, such as the brain, heart, and muscles, and less to those body parts that can get along on short supplies for at least the duration of the emergency—the skin, gut, and kidneys, for example.

These responses are so sudden and usually so profound that most people have had the experience of an overwhelming physical reaction when they are frightened, angry, or threatened in any way. The skin cools as the blood vessels constrict to send the blood elsewhere, and the eyes dilate in the presence of adrenalin flow. Many people feel their heart race or pound when they sense danger as the heart immediately steps up its work. The mouth dries as adrenalin slows the flow of saliva. Most important, all of the senses are heightened as a result of sympathetic nervous system stimulation. Prepared for fight or flight by these circulating sympathetic substances, the individual sees and hears better; he experiences a sudden surge of strength and his responses are quickened and acute.

But this heightened state of awareness exacts a cost. The heart is working much harder than usual to produce the added blood flow needed to power the sympathetic nervous system response. If there is underlying coronary artery disease and a part of the heart muscle cannot obtain the increased blood supply it needs to perform this extra work, this part of the heart may become ischemic. Deprived of the blood flow it requires and the oxygen carried by the blood, the heart may signal with the pain of angina; if ignored, oxygen starvation may lead to even more serious problems. It is primarily for this reason that people with coronary artery disease are counseled to avoid stress as much as possible and to avoid placing undue demands on their heart. A heart that is already damaged by an infarct or by a coronary artery that is known to be impaired by atherosclerotic disease should not be taxed by the extra work demanded by sympathetic nervous system activity.

EFFECTS OF SYMPATHETIC NERVOUS SYSTEM STIMULATION

Adrenalin and nonadrenalin, lifesavers in an emergency, also have marked effects on the blood pressure and can raise it to dangerously high levels. The rise in blood pressure, sometimes quite precipitous and often sustained for a significant period of time, may play a part in the sudden onset of chest pain or the heart attack that sometimes occurs during acute stress. This sudden rise in blood pressure may also play a role in the development of stroke or cerebrovascular accident.

Another danger in the sudden onset of sympathetic nervous system activity has to do with its role in possibly stimulating an abnormal rhythm in the heart. Arrhythmias of this kind are usually manifest as rapid rhythms, but they may appear as ventricular ectopic beats (skipped beats) that can, on occasion, degenerate into life-threatening ventricular fibrillation. Fortunately, this is not a common occurrence but it can happen in patients with underlying heart abnormalities.

Stress may also affect the heart by way of the elevations of serum lipid levels that accompany sympathetic nervous system activity. Cholesterol tends to be high under constant stress; triglyceride levels rise during acute stress as does the level of free fatty acids in the bloodstream. These serum lipid elevations may trigger an arrhythmia, or may at least provide a clue to the method by which stress produces cardiac damage. Chronic stress, producing chronic lipid elevation, may also play a role in the formation of atherosclerosis, although this has not yet been clinically documented and may prove to be of only secondary importance.

Another bodily response to stress provides still another clue —and raises still more questions. It has been known for years that sympathetic stimulation, or even the administration of artificial sympathetic neural transmitters, increases the tendency of the blood to clot. (The acute rise in serum lipids caused by sympathetic nervous system activity may also play a role in thrombotic events known to affect the heart.) Although this is an important defense mechanism—if one is about to go into battle where the risk of injury is great, rapid blood clotting would have enormous survival value—its inappropriate occurrence in the bloodstream can lead to life-threatening thrombotic events.

But as noted many times before, the situations that induce stress in modern man are only rarely of this nature. In most cases twentieth-century man calls up these substances to handle battles of quite a different sort. The blood is prepared to clot in case of injury, probably by way of the action of the adrenalin and noradrenalin on the platelets themselves, because the sympathetic nervous system has been conditioned by generations of evolutionary selection to perceive the possibility of bleeding to death as a real risk. But when this action is chronic and sympathetic stimulation is called up chronically and inappropriately to increase the tendency of the platelets to aggregate, the stage is set for the occurrence of a damaging and possibly life-threatening clot.

The site of the clot, of course, determines the nature of the damage. A clot or thrombosis in the brain will result in a stroke, while a clot which blocks a coronary vessel may produce a heart attack. In other cases a clot appearing in a large vessel and doing little or no damage at that site may break off and travel to a more vital body part—the lungs, heart, or brain—and cause serious problems there. Other things also influence the development of a clot but there is no question that sympathetic stimulation increases the tendency of the platelets to aggregate, stress in this way contributing to a serious physiological problem.

EFFECTS OF THE PARASYMPATHETIC NERVOUS SYSTEM

Another bodily effect of stress has to do with its role in a sudden inappropriate firing of the parasympathetic nervous system. You will recall that the parasympathetic nervous system maintains the normal vegetative processes at normal levels when the body is at rest, lowering the heart rate during sleep to keep everything working efficiently, for example. If it fires inappropriately, however, there is a marked slowing of the heart rate, occasionally almost to a standstill. This inappropriate parasympathetic response may lower the blood pressure to a level that does not provide enough blood to perfuse the brain. If it continues, the slowed heart rate and dropped blood pressure can deny the heart the blood it needs to perfuse its own coronaries, resulting in cardiac ischemia or starvation. If the parasympathetic impulses are strong and if there is an underlying abnormality in the heart, an arrhythmia may result. Usually of the slow variety and usually having to do with heart block, these slow rhythms may favor the emergence of abnormal ectopic beats or, even more serious, life-threatening ventricular fibrillation.

Interestingly, the abrupt slowing caused by inappropriate parasympathetic release is related to another facet of stress, the "giving-up" reaction. Researchers have been puzzled when experimental animals die unexpectedly in the course of stress studies. When the animals are examined no physical cause of death can be determined and researchers conclude that they have been stressed to the point where they just give up. We do not really understand why this happens or exactly how it is related to coronary death in humans, but we do know that some people die of despair—and that this is just another aspect of stress. Physiologically, the vagus nerve is probably somehow involved but it is also probably true that in man there is a great psychophysiological component in the equation that may explain why some people survive great stress while others succumb to it at once.

Of a far less serious nature is the marked emotional response frequently seen in people with strong vasomotor activity. Younger people sometimes react to the emotion of seeing a pop singer, for example, by fainting, an effect of parasympathetic stimulation. Fainting is a parasympathetic response frequently preceded by symptoms of dizziness, irritability, loss of attention, and a cold sweat which is related to the drop in blood pressure. When the blood pressure and heart rate drop to the point where there is not enough cardiac output to reach the brain, the individual faints. Usually just lying flat on the floor restores blood flow to the head and after a moment or two the patient revives, somewhat weakened but with no lasting damage.

If this vasomotor syncope takes place in someone with heart disease, however, a strong parasympathetic response induced by stress can trigger a more severe problem. There may be enough oxygen starvation to cause some loss of myocardial tissue—a heart attack—or this extreme hypotension can disturb the rhythm of the heart, causing an arrhythmia. A strong parasympathetic response to stress, usually inappropriate, can in these ways result in sudden death. This is again a rare effect of acute stress that is usually emotional in nature.

The more chronic effects of parasympathetic nervous system activity are usually related to the vegetative systems concerned with visceral tone. Most of its effects are seen in the gastrointestinal tract; increased parasympathetic tone leads to the oversecretion of enzymes and acids in the stomach and may play a part in the development of ulcers. The increase in parasympathetic neural tone is also suspected of increasing the activity of the large bowel, possibly causing psychogenic diarrhea (the well-known "nervous stomach"), and possibly, although this is not clear, playing a role in the development of the symptoms of ulcerative colitis.

THE EFFECTS OF STEROID HORMONES

The body also responds to stress by secreting, or hypersecreting, hormones, the adrenal steroids. These cortisonelike hormones secreted by another part of the adrenal gland in the presence of stress are another survival mechanism that acts to moderate the body's response to infection or trauma and to strengthen its reactions.

In the last thirty years, Dr. Hans Selye, working with his group in Canada, has conducted extensive experiments that have shown that the presence of large amounts of steroid hormones tends to sensitize the heart to the effects of stress. In experimental animals subjected to a great deal of stress or in animals injected with steroids, Selye has observed patches of loss of tissue and damage to the heart muscle. The exact physiologic relationship to the role of stress in human heart disease is still unknown, but there is an interesting clue in the fact that the levels of circulating steroid hormones go up in people who are under prolonged stress as well as in those who are undergoing the particular stress of myocardial infarction.

Chronic physical stress in humans is known to elevate the production of steroid hormones; whether this is also the case in emotional stress and whether the levels achieved by the inappropriate secretion of steroid hormones are sufficient to cause genuine cardiac damage is still not known. It is significant, too, that these hormones in abundance, probably more than would be secreted during stress, will also cause salt retention that eventually elevates the blood pressure, another negative action which may be inflicted by stress on the human body.

Stress also acts on the heart through its effects on the body's normal reparative function. Chronic and acute stress markedly reduce the ability of the tissues to repair themselves. The loss of sleep that many people experience when they are under great emotional stress can itself lead to a breaking down of the normal reparative processes. People who chronically get insufficient sleep simply cannot tolerate stress well. They respond more actively and irrationally to stress than does a rested individual. Everyone has had the experience of snapping out in tension at something that under normal circumstances would scarcely rank as an annoyance. Laboratory studies have shown definite emotional and psychophysiological changes in patients who are fatigued.

PSYCHOSOCIAL DETERMINANTS OF STRESS

People who have studied stress in modern man note that the subject is like a labyrinth, with many twists and turns in what was thought to be a relatively straight road. The businessman who makes it to the top, for example, was always thought to be a prime candidate for a coronary. Traditionally, the executive suite was considered the site of more heart attacks than any other location.

But further studies indicate that it is actually those in middle management positions who suffer the most premature heart disease. "Getting it" from both sides so to speak, from their bosses above as well as from the workers beneath them, and unable to directly affect the outcome of their efforts, men in middle level positions appear to have more heart attacks than those who are fixed at either end of the executive spectrum.

Actually, the whole concept of financial and social mobility is operant here. In rigidly structured societies, where men are expected to achieve no more than their fathers did before them, premature heart disease is not the problem that it is in more "democratic" countries. Life may not be easy in the so-called backward nations where this situation exists today, and there is no question that it was not easy generations ago in this country when great forces were at work to keep men at their known station in life, but it should be recognized that the freedom to move upward exacts a great cost. Every man is expected today to do better than his father did, and the need to climb ever higher on the ladder of success is implicit in everything we do. The opportunities are there and the implication is that those who do not succeed just have not tried hard enough. If you do not "make it" in a mobile and success-oriented society, you are made to feel that it is no one's fault but your own. Stress is thus a component of the success syndrome. There is enormous pressure to succeed, to make it big; disappointment and stress remain for those who fail.

In these highly competitive roles, then, men endure an enormous amount of stress. The pressure to earn more money, the pressure to maintain a decent standard of living, and the struggle to achieve security when it is difficult to conceptualize one's role in a complex technology are some of the strains that not infrequently lead to organic illnesses such as ulcers, colitis, allergic phenomena, asthmatic attacks, and, of course, heart attacks.

STRESS AND THE JOB

Another of the many blind alleys we grope in when we discuss present-day stress concerns the estrangement of many workers, at all levels, from the product of their work. The satisfaction that a craftsman feels when he completes an object and the security that even the poorest farmer could develop by harvesting his own crops are for the most part denied to workers of today. Factory workers who spend tedious hours at one small fraction of a task have rightly begun to demand a restructuring of their working conditions. Although their demands probably had little to do with health considerations, what they ask is the sense of satisfaction that comes from achieving a finished product, a security that is denied to them in the present setup.

The situation is exactly the same among white-collar workers. Many patients trying to rush their convalescence from a heart attack confide their real fears to me: they are anxious to return to work before someone realizes that their job can be eliminated with little or no loss to the company. Far removed from the end product of their efforts, workers today express their insecurity in many ways; discontent, alcoholism, ulcers, and heart attacks are but a few.

The speed with which industries come and go today contributes to the stress that is experienced by many workers. Trained to perform a highly technical job, skilled engineers, for example, suddenly found that the aerospace industry had almost gone the way of the blacksmith shop. Less highly trained people, often large numbers of them, often wake up one day to find that a machine has been programmed to do their job—faster, cheaper, more accurately, and around the clock.

This produces genuine stress and the human machine is not programmed to take it without great cost to the system. And humans age; even the brightest young man experiences the familiar knot in the stomach when a still younger man eyes his desk hungrily.

It is no wonder that alcoholism, instability, and stress pervade the working environment today. Independence among workers is all but unknown. The loner, struggling by himself toward an impossible goal, is little more than a myth in a highly developed society like ours where everyone, and everything, depends on others. Even top men must answer to someone, and there are few functioning human beings who do not know the insecurity and stress of depending on someone else for their livelihood.

Other aspects of job stress have also been studied, with sadly impressive results. A survey of coronary heart disease among American physicians revealed that the more "stressful" specialties of anesthesiology and general practice exacted a far higher toll in terms of disease than did the "easier" specialties of pathology and dermatology. Another study of young men with heart disease disclosed that almost all of them had occupied positions of great responsibility that were frequently associated with emotional strain.

STRESS AND THE CITY

The urban environment itself is suspected of causing no small amount of stress. Noisy, crowded, frustrating, and sometimes dangerous—it would be hard to depict the American city as anything but stressful. Studies have indicated that big city dwellers are in an almost constant state of being "up"—catecholamines flowing and the heart working to provide the extra power they need to stay afloat in a hostile environment. In big cities the stimulation is constant and, although there are those who would argue that it breeds creativity and achievement in many fields, there are others who would say that the price is too high. For New Yorkers and other urban dwellers have far more than their share of stress-related problems. It is no accident that there are more psychiatrists in New York (and more psychotherapists in Los Angeles) than anywhere else in the world. Ulcers, hypertension, psychiatric problems, and heart attacks all appear with more frequency under the stress of big city life.

Many researchers have traveled to the small town of Roseto in central Pennsylvania to try to learn why the town is relatively immune to premature heart disease. For years Roseto townspeople, mostly Italian and many overweight on a good diet of pasta and rich native foods, appeared to beat the odds. Their life expectancy was ten to twelve years longer than the nation's in general and the rate of heart disease, especially among younger men, was lower than would be expected.

Since there were few objective differences between Roseto and neighboring towns, early research concluded that the fortunate people of Roseto were protected from heart disease by the remarkably supportive environment of their close-knit community. In a town where everyone knew everybody else and where interrelated families created an unusual kind of security, it was almost impossible to know either poverty or the stress produced by its threat. Most people grew up in Roseto knowing that in one way or another, they would never starve.

But a more recent look indicates that today's generation of Roseto townspeople is no different from any other small town dwellers. Death from heart attacks in men under fifty, almost un-known thirty years ago, is not now so rare and life expectancy in Roseto is similar to that in other communities. Some investigators who have studied the town extensively believe that an ever-rising standard of living has eroded much of the supportive environment enjoyed by earlier generations. As certain members of the community have become rich, pressure on others has developed in terms of personal drive for success and aspirations for their children. Dr. John Bruhn, one of the researchers who has studied Roseto, commented: "The town where people lived longer than most anywhere else and where love of family and closeness of community made them nearly immune to heart attack is feeling the subtle effects of what happens when the American dream comes true." This stress of upward mobility may be the straw that breaks the camel's back in terms of heart disease.

THE "NORMAL" STRESS OF LIVING

Stress, of course, is everywhere. Even so routine a matter as the domestic status, married or otherwise, appears to have some effect on a person's health. Single people—widowed, divorced, or never married—suffer significantly more illness, especially heart-related problems, than do married folk. The married relationship, even apparently when it is not ideal, seems to provide the support-ive environment that many people need to remain healthy. The figures are worse for men than for women. Men who have a spouse appear to enjoy measurably improved health and longer life.

Several researchers have sought to quantify the impact of normal stress. By assigning numbers to, or ranking the various strains that most humans are heir to, this field of research—partly in the field of psychology, partly in medicine—attempts to identify those who are at especially high risk for heart attacks or mental breakdowns or other manifestations of stress which are dealt with incompetently. Their thesis, very simply put, is that "a cluster of life events requiring change in the individual's accustomed way of life is significantly associated with the onset of disease." According to this and other studies, within two years of a life event certain susceptible people can expect to experience some mental or physi-cal symptoms.

Dr. Thomas Holmes, a psychiatrist at the University of Washington, has devised an instrument called the Schedule of Recent Experiences (SRE), a listing of life experiences which have been ranked numerically, shown in Table 7–1. The people who participated in the development of the SRE were asked to rate each life event in terms of its social readjustment—social readjustment being defined as "the intensity and length of time necessary to accommodate to a life event, regardless of the desirability of this event."

This definition is important because according to these studies it is the individual's *ability to adjust* to changes in his life that determines his response to stress. Thus, death of a spouse ranks first in terms of adjustment required, divorce second, marital separation third—with a jail term running fourth. It is interesting that life events relating to marriage occupy the first rank of positions, since we have already noted that people who are single, for any reason, appear to have a higher disease rate than others. At the end of the list of forty-three life events are such things as changes in eating or sleeping habits, vacations, Christmas, and minor violations of the law. Follow-up studies confirmed that most American adults would rank life events in this or similar order. The list developed by Drs. Holmes and Rahe is reproduced on page 155. Each life event is assigned a numerical value of stress, and the authors suggest that when a total score greater than 300 is reached in a single year, the chances of suffering significant physical illness is great.

STRESS AND SUDDEN DEATH

Dr. George Engel, of the Strong Memorial Hospital in Rochester, New York, has investigated the phenomenon of sudden death following acute psychological stress. Of the 170 people who died suddenly and unexpectedly following such stress, three were children under the age of ten and four were teenagers. Most of the men who died in these emotionally stressful situations were between the ages of forty-five and fifty-five years old, while women were older, seventy to seventy-five years old.

A remarkable series of accounts of death, all of Dr. Engel's material relates to people who were found on examination or autopsy to have no actual physical cause of death. He concluded that, although most died following situations of various kinds of losses ("on the impact of the collapse or death of a close person, during

THE SOCIAL READJUSTMENT RATING SCALE

Life Event	Mean Value
1. Death of spouse	100
2. Divorce	73
3. Marital separation from mate	65
4. Detention in jail or other institution	63
5. Death of a close family member	63
6. Major personal injury or illness	53
7. Marriage	50
8. Being fired at work	47
9. Marital reconciliation with mate	45
10. Retirement from work	45
11. Major change in the health or behavior of a family member	44
12. Pregnancy	40
13. Sexual difficulties	39
14. Gaining a new family member (e.g., through birth, adoption, oldster moving in, etc.)	39
15. Major business readjustment (e.g., merger, reorganization, bankruptcy, etc.)	39
16. Major change in financial state (e.g., a lot worse off or a lot better off than usual)	38
17. Death of a close friend	37
18. Changing to a different line of work	36
19. Major change in the number of arguments with spouse (e.g., either a lot more or a lot less than usual regarding child-rearing, personal habits, etc.)	35
20. Taking on a mortgage greater than $10,000 (e.g., purchasing a home, business, etc.)	31
21. Foreclosure on a mortgage or loan	30
22. Major change in responsibilities at work (e.g., promotion, demotion, lateral transfer)	29
23. Son or daughter leaving home (e.g., marriage, attending college, etc.)	29
24. In-law troubles	29
25. Outstanding personal achievement	28
26. Wife beginning or ceasing work outside the home	26
27. Beginning or ceasing formal schooling	26
28. Major change in living conditions (e.g., building a new home, remodeling, deterioration of home or neighborhood)	25
29. Revision of personal habits (dress, manners, associations, etc.)	24
30. Troubles with the boss	23

Life Event	Mean Value
31. Major change in working hours or conditions	20
32. Change in residence	20
33. Changing to a new school	20
34. Major change in usual type and/or amount of recreation	19
35. Major change in church activities (e.g., a lot more or a lot less than usual)	19
36. Major change in social activities (e.g., clubs, dancing, movies, visiting, etc.)	18
37. Taking on a mortgage or loan less than $10,000 (e.g., purchasing a car, TV, freezer, etc.)	17
38. Major change in sleeping habits (a lot more or a lot less sleep, or change in part of day when asleep)	16
39. Major change in number of family get-togethers (e.g., a lot more or a lot less than usual)	15
40. Major change in eating habits (a lot more or a lot less food intake, or very different meal hours or surroundings)	15
41. Vacation	13
42. Christmas	12
43. Minor violation of the law (e.g., traffic tickets, jaywalking, disturbing the peace, etc.)	11

Reprinted with permission from *Journal of Psychosomatic Research II*, 213-218: T. H. Holmes and R. H. Rahe, The Social Readjustment Rating Scale; 1967, Pergamon Press, Ltd.

acute grief, on threat of loss of a close person, during mourning or on an anniversary of a death"), or as a reaction to personal danger or threats ("loss of status or self-esteem, personal danger, or threat of injury"), some died almost as a relief reaction ("after the danger is over, and [following] reunion, triumph, or happy ending"). More men died following loss of self-esteem or an abrupt change in status (as would occur in the case of business reverses), but more women died in relation to grief or mourning. A situation of danger appeared to affect men more than it did women.

Several common denominators appeared in Dr. Engel's study. What he called the lethal life situations appeared to involve events that the victims felt they could not ignore. Overwhelmed by events perceived to be beyond their control or mastery, many victims were felt to give up or to indulge in frantic ineffective activity, the same responses often noted in laboratory animals who are used in stress experimentation. Unable to fight or to escape and feeling themselves to be in totally impossible situations, some people responded by suddenly dying. But it was also noted that some people died suddenly on the anniversary of a death or mourning while others died after the danger had passed. And, perhaps most poignant of all, some sudden deaths occurred at a moment of triumph or success—the so-called "happy ending" deaths.

THE CORONARY-PRONE PERSONALITY

It should be apparent by now that human beings react to stress with bodily responses that sometimes predispose to illness or death; the data are conclusive and overwhelming. But after we know this—that events both good and bad demand personal adjustment of varying difficulty—where do we go from here? Specifically in terms of heart disease and other life-threatening illnesses, what do we do? One approach to the problem of how to live with stress is to locate those people whose personalities give some indication of being unable to respond without untoward or dangerous physiologic effects.

In terms of prevention of heart attacks, the most fruitful area of personality research seems to lie in the identification of the coronary-prone individual. To identify the behavior patterns most strongly associated with the occurrence of premature heart disease seems a reasonable route toward its prevention.

The distinctive personality of the coronary-prone individual was recognized many years ago. Dr. William Osler, lecturing in 1897 on angina pectoris, described its typical victim as a "keen and ambitious man, the indicator of whose engines is always set full speed ahead." Years later, in 1958, Dr. Henry Russek, a New York cardiologist, became interested in what he considered the lethal interaction of stress with other known risk factors (smoking, diet, and heredity) in young adults. In describing the usual behavior of young men with coronary disease, Russek noted that they frequently felt great emotional strain in their work and experienced guilt and restlessness during what was supposed to be leisure time. The drive and intense ambition of the coronary-prone personality and a peculiar lack of satisfaction with the results of their efforts have also been noted by other investigators.

It is easy to see how the cumulative effect of these attitudes are in themselves stressful; superimposed on an individual who probably smokes too much, eats erratically, and who certainly has little time for either rest or regular exercise, they may spell trouble. Russek's work presents evidence that a high fat diet interacts with stress to form a most lethal combination, and he presents evidence that the other risk factors work with stress in much the same catalytic way.

THE TYPE A CORONARY-PRONE PERSONALITY

At the Brunn Institute in San Francisco, Drs. Meyer Friedman and Ray Rosenman conduct ongoing studies concerned with the identification of the coronary-prone personality. Early in 1959, these cardiologists reported some distinctive behavior patterns among their coronary patients. When they sought to interview people who had had heart attacks, even those who were still hospitalized, they noticed a preoccupation with time and its passage that struck them as significant. Many of the coronary patients the doctors talked to lacked the patience to listen closely; they finished sentences for the interviewers or answered questions before they were asked. Along with this rather obvious impatience with time, many coronary patients exhibited other distinctive personality characteristics that Rosenman and Friedman came to call the "Type A Personality."

In one of their early studies, reported in the *Journal of the American Medical Association* in 1959, they gave the classic description of what has come to be known as the coronary-prone personality: "an intense, sustained drive to achieve self-selected but usually poorly defined goals ... profound inclination and eagerness to compete ... persistent desire for recognition and advancement ... continuous involvement in multiple and diverse functions constantly subject to time restrictions (deadlines) ... habitual propensity to accelerate the rate of execution of many physical and mental functions ... and extraordinary mental and physical alertness."

In the same study, Rosenman and Friedman noted that "a person was adjudged as exhibiting completely developed behavior pattern A if he exhibited various signs indicative of its presence, including excessively rapid body movements, tense facial and body musculature, explosive conversational intonations, hand or teeth clenching, excessive unconscious gesturing, and a general air of impatience, and if he admitted his sustained drive, competitiveness, and a necessity to accelerate many activities and was aware of a chronic sense of urgency in daily living. . . ."

The Type B personality pattern was essentially the converse of Type A and was characterized by "a relative absence of drive, ambition, sense of urgency, desire to compete, involvement in deadlines. . . ." The typical Type B man, in contrast to the harried Type A, "sat relaxedly, moved slowly and calmly, exhibited no muscular tension, spoke slowly, rarely indulged in tense gestures, exhibited no impatience and denied even moderate drive or ambition, shunned competition, avoided involvement in deadlines, and felt no sense of urgency."

In the 1959 report, usually considered the first of the series, Type A men were noted to work harder and longer (an average of fifty-two hours per week) and to smoke more than other less driven men. The investigators noted that Type A men had higher average serum cholesterol levels than Type B men, and also had a strikingly higher incidence of arcus senilis, a change in the border of the cornea of the eye frequently associated with premature aging and atherosclerosis. There was also more rapid blood clotting among Type A men.

Most important was the finding of increased incidence of coronary artery disease. Far more Type A men, twenty-three of the eighty-three subjects, had signs of premature coronary artery disease and all of the overt cases were found in men who had been identified at the outset as having the fully developed behavior pattern—that is, the Complete Type A Man. This was further corroborated by the finding that the three cases of coronary artery disease found among the Type B men were in those individuals who showed some Type A characteristics, that is, who were considered incompletely developed Type Bs.

In commenting on their findings, the authors noted that since both groups ate approximately the same diet the differences in cholesterol levels indicated that a factor other than diet was clearly operant. But they further suggested that the "lethalness of high fat intake for man apparently depends on an *interplay* with other important factors."

In later studies these same researchers attempted to identify the mechanisms through which Type A behavior patterns increased both serum cholesterol levels and the incidence of clinical coronary artery disease. Further analysis of their data suggested that Type A personalities had a heart attack rate that was *two-and-one-half times* that of their less driven colleagues; in younger men under the age of fifty the ratio appeared to be even higher.

Two years later, in 1961, Rosenman and Friedman reported essentially the same results in a study of 257 women, a group which included thirty-nine nuns. Type A women, both pre- and postmenopausal, "smoked more cigarettes, drank more alcohol, had a far higher incidence of arcus senilis, much higher serum cholesterol levels, and, among the premenopausal subjects, a significantly faster clotting time." These findings suggested that many of these things are associative rather than causative factors; that is, they appear along with, rather than as causes of, certain patterns of health and behavior.

It was significant, however, that Type A women had *four times* the incidence of coronary heart disease along with an increased frequency of high blood pressure. Again the researchers noted that, although serum cholesterol levels may affect the development of atherosclerotic plaque, it may be the individual's behavior patterns that determine the outcome in terms of health, or its obverse of heart disease and death.

Later studies examined the biochemical characteristics of proven Type A and B personalities. Again Type A persons were shown to have significantly higher cholesterol and triglyceride levels and also exhibited a higher insulin response to glucose. Since these elevations are associated with the occurrence of coronary heart disease, the researchers looked for still other biochemical differences between the two groups. They also noted that Type A excreted more norepinephrine, the chemical mediator of the sympathetic nervous system, *during working hours of the day,* than did Type B individuals.

A more ominous finding, reported in the September, 1973 issue of the *Journal of the American Medical Association,* is that the Type A personality was found with significantly greater frequency among those who died suddenly as a result of cardiac dysfunction.

STRESS AND ITS RELATION TO HEART DISEASE

The effort to identify the coronary-prone personality continues in laboratories all over the world. Although much of the work derives from Rosenman's and Friedman's early studies, it should be noted that there are not many people who would be considered either pure Type A or pure Type B. Most people have been found to have characteristics of both types, but there are still measurable differences in the heart disease rate between those who are predominantly Type A and those who are predominantly Type B.

There is no question that the individual's response to his environment and his personality play a great role in determining the probability of his developing heart disease. In England, Dr. H. E. S. Pearson and his group interviewed a large cohort of men concerning their attitudes toward home, work, leisure activities, and social status. The interviews were far-ranging and dealt with attitudes in general rather than with hard, specific questions. It was noteworthy that, although the interviewers did not know which men had coronary artery disease, they accurately reported a significantly higher incidence of stressful response from those men who proved to have a clinical history of heart disease than from those who did not.

Drs. Henry I. Russek and Burton Zohman, in this country, ranked men on the basis of four of the known risk factors for coronary heart disease: cholesterol levels, smoking, heredity, and stress. They found that stress correlated best with the prior incidence of myocardial infarction—90 percent of those with coronary disease ranking positive for stress. Among the disease-free men used as controls, a far smaller number exhibited stressful traits.

Other researchers are looking into the correlation between elevated uric acid levels indicative of gout and the incidence of heart disease. They seem to be associated to some extent, but the interesting finding that gout is also correlated with high intelligence and achievement may provide one of the links between the ambitious and success-oriented Type A individual and his risk of heart attack.

THE MANAGEMENT OF STRESS

The central question is, of course, how to manage the coronary-prone personality, how to live with stress. While there are many unanswered questions, the experience of many years suggests that therapeutic measures must be instituted even while the solutions to basic matters are still being sought.

Personality is an attitude, a way of relating to one's peers and surroundings. Attitudes are not easily changed, but I want to assure every reader that many of their destructive aspects can be altered. People who have had a heart attack, for example, often change from a pure Type A to a moderated Type B+, an important and valuable modification. It is regrettable that so often this is done in the coronary care unit, but many patients learn there to consider the important things—life and death itself—rather than the daily minor crises that have for so long kept them in a state of almost constant stress.

But apart from this extreme, which presents an agonizing but "easy" means of changing behavior, what else can be done to alter the personality and possibly slow the development of atherosclerosis in the coronary-prone personality? What can be done to possibly prevent the heart attack he appears headed for?

Most physicians agree that it is vital to consider behavior patterns in any patient who already exhibits one or more of the known risk factors. People with hypertension, diabetes, and elevated cholesterol levels as well as those with a family history of heart disease should be counseled in terms of the "coronary-proneness" of their personality.

Thus it is important that patients know that their risk of heart disease, already increased by the presence of one or more of the known risk factors, is exacerbated by typical Type A behavior. The associational relationship is strong: high-strung people smoke more and their impatience with time and dissatisfaction with their own efforts tend to raise their blood pressure with depressing frequency. When they exercise they bring to what should be a leisure activity the same intensity and aggressiveness that marks their other activities. As a matter of fact, some physicians believe that men over thirty-five should approach competitive sports such as tennis singles and handball cautiously, if at all, since this kind of activity seems to bring out Type A behavior in everyone, often with deleterious results.

Counseling those who are coronary-prone, then, must begin with the modification of the controllable risk factors. Even mild hypertension should be followed and treated, usually over a long period of time. Cholesterol levels should be checked often and appropriate steps taken by everyone to reduce fat intake. It is further evidence of the relationship between stress and the other risk factors that blood pressure and cholesterol levels can sometimes be used to indicate the effectiveness of efforts aimed at moderating the personality. Even as the patient struggles with drugs or dietary treatment, the destructive power of Type A sometimes essentially negates any other therapy. Dr. Friedman concludes: "After over fifteen years of seeing and treating coronary-prone subjects, as well as already victimized coronary patients, we suspect that, *if Type A behavior pattern when present is not altered,* other forms of treatment directed against either the first or a recurrent coronary heart attack are relatively inadequate and disappointing."

Beyond these clinical steps, the prudent man must achieve some insight into the nature of his personality. For some people just knowing the cost exacted by their stressful reactions is enough. Facing the question, "why am I killing myself like this?", some fortunate folk are able to change their behavior, to reevaluate their goals, and come to some understanding of the role of time and achievement in their lives. For others, a mild tranquilizer is occasionally helpful. These drugs are often effective and are prescribed to aid in the control of health-consuming emotions. They are relatively safe if taken under a physician's guidance in the proper dosage and can help to tide a harried individual over an exceptionally difficult period.

DEALING WITH DAY-TO-DAY STRESS

The goal of any treatment for stress is to free the patient of his virtual enslavement to the demands of time and his excessive response to the emotional strains of living. What is needed is a standard against which to judge a person's responses. As we have seen, some people react to the stress of life in a state of almost constant agitation. Obsessed with the passage of time, they are always "up." But if these classic Type A's attempted some small scale personal psychology, they would see that crises have a way of grading themselves from serious to whimsical and that life requires judgment of what is important and what is not.

Some questions are probably in order. Are your responses appropriate to the situation? Is your haste real or are you just in the habit of rushing everywhere? Think about your most recent rage. Was it worth it? Was it important? What were you really angry about? Overall, are you tense most of the time? How do you feel about yourself in general?

The questions could go on and on, but the important thing is to determine those situations over which you have some control from those in which you have little or none. How real is the crisis and how much can you do to affect it? Take a moment to consider whether it is realistic to expend your valuable psychic energy on it. It is not easy to make these judgments, but I can assure you that it is the kind of control that might just pay off in the fight against psychogenic disease.

The people who successfully control their responses to stress begin by realizing that their responses to stress often have little relation to the reality of the situation. That is, frequently it is not the actual stress itself but the attitude of the individual toward the situation that produces hazardous physiological changes. The following simple exercise shows the futility of most stress. What was your major concern a year ago? What troubled you most six months ago? Most people cannot even remember what was troubling them as recently as two weeks ago. The events that caused so much grief a year earlier usually mean little today. (Genuine loss is always recalled, of course, but we refer here to the erroneous judgment of transient or imaginary stress.) If you cannot recall, or if you dimly remember that a year ago you lost a night's sleep over something of really transitory importance, then you are on to what we mean by an unnecessarily stressful response to the quite ordinary strain of daily living. Looking back it is easy to see your overreaction; what is not easy is to put today's troubles into the same perspective.

The real challenge is to develop the same detachment and objectivity with regard to today's problems that are so easily seen in regard to those that happened some time ago. And a comforting by-product in terms of work to be done is that the objective individual usually accomplishes more, since hysteria and emotional stress are usually counterproductive. It is probably helpful to develop a productive attitude toward worry itself. Only if it really helps to worry—if the individual is actually aided toward a solution by the act of worrying itself—should he indulge in this usually wasteful activity. Genuine wisdom, I am convinced, lies in knowing the difference between those situations where worry is helpful from those where it is only an impediment. To spend a great deal of time and psychic energy worrying about situations that one cannot affect is not only a futile waste of time and emotion but also possibly deleterious. Remember, the attitude toward your problem is far more important, usually, than the problem itself.

A corollary to this, especially for the classic Type A who takes little pleasure or satisfaction in his achievements, is to develop tolerance and patience and a genuine appreciation for one's efforts. It is no accident that for some time the best-selling book in the United States was a slim volume that entreated everyone to be his own best friend. Too many people are saddled with a chronic dissatisfaction with themselves and the product of their labors. Forever unsatisfied, they experience great stress that could easily be avoided by a small dose of self-approval taken with liberal quantities of acceptance. "I did my best." No man can do more or say more in his own behalf.

BASIC HUMAN NEEDS: A REFUGE

In addition to the vital matter of the attitude with which one comes to regard living, there are at least three ways to better tolerate the stress of daily living. The first, absolutely essential, is that each individual must have a refuge. Everyone, especially those who are experiencing the particular strains of the middle years, must have a place where they can escape the real problems of the day. For some lucky men, just returning to the home and family is helpful and supportive. When they are fortunate enough to have a wife who works at creating this nonthreatening ambience, some men are able to forget the problems they face in the course of the normal day. The home then becomes an energizer as well as a sanctuary; they can relax and enjoy the renewing strength of a warm and pleasant refuge.

Since it is mostly men who suffer premature heart attacks, I must stress that women should understand that the desirable home is a refuge, an escape from the sometimes intolerable reality of the working world. A wife should try to create the kind of surroundings that are as supportive and health-giving and as remote from the working world as is possible. Only if she is actively seeking illness, despair, and widowhood should she spend her time pushing and criticizing, tearing down the defenses that every man needs to survive in the modern jungle.

The household should be organized so that, when the husband comes home, he is not immediately bombarded with a long recital of the problems of the day. These can be trotted out later, after a drink perhaps or a quiet period during which the "old man" is allowed the luxury of catching his breath. Most men have considerable stress in the course of a working day. They should not be burdened or annoyed by the turmoil, either physical or mental, of housekeeping. A woman should listen well, sympathizing with daily problems, and giving, in every way, the support that only a woman can. And if a man prefers not to discuss his problems, that's all right too.

In some situations it is not possible to create a refuge of this kind, for it is the home itself that causes stress, and the working place becomes the refuge. Sad, because in these situations some men succeed in killing themselves by contriving never to leave the office. Too often they work themselves to death in an effort to get away from the stress of home.

Other men, in other situations, find that they can relax only by getting out one or two evenings a week. This should never be permitted to become a matter of contention; if a man must go out once or twice a week, it should be understood that his need is for a refuge. Too often, unfortunately, the need for a refuge is not fulfilled in a healthful manner; some men overindulge in alcohol or drugs to create a destructive kind of refuge from their problems.

Any healthful escape is absolutely necessary to the well-being of the individual, especially when it is used to counter the effects of chronic stress on the heart. Thus it is vital that vacations be used effectively. On the long vacation, the two weeks or a month each year that the family takes to get away, it is essential that the father, who usually endures the most stress at other times, try to get the best rest. For this reason I consider a vacation where dad drives the family across the country a poor choice for most working men. A rest by the sea or some time in one lovely resort strikes me as a much better vacation for a man who works hard the remainder of the year.

To creatively use the weekend as the short vacation it was no doubt intended to be is also helpful. Unfortunately most people use the weekend to catch up with all the chores left undone during the week. This is absolutely wrong. From antiquity it has been known that at least one day a week must be set aside for rest, to retire emotionally and physically from the strains of the week. Rather than working or catching up, at least one day each week should be set aside by every working man to do exactly what he chooses to do. And he should decide in advance that he is not going to do anything he does not want to do. Some men will choose to sleep as late as they wish, read the paper at leisure, and relax for the remainder of the day. Others will choose to play golf or take apart the family car if they find this relaxing; one wonderful old gentleman tells me that he spends at least an hour, every Saturday afternoon in a warm bathtub, a marvelously relaxing experience. Some men enjoy a two-hour nap in the afternoon. The important thing is that this time be considered his inviolably. If his wife wants him to go shopping or to put up the storm windows, he must point out that this one day is his and that she must work out a different plan.

I believe it is exceedingly important that a man use this short one-day-a-week vacation to retire from stress, to recharge his batteries, and to regain the vantage that allows him to look with detachment upon all the things that were so stressful during the week. In this way some insight can be gained, and most men will feel that they are once again in control of their lives. Renewed in vigor, they are better able to handle the problems that surely lie ahead.

Because it is medically true that many more men than women are victims of heart attacks, especially at younger ages, the preceding discussion emphasizes the wife's role in alleviating stress. But women are subject to stress and coronary heart disease, too, so men are well advised to show the same understanding for the problems of their wives.

BASIC HUMAN NEEDS: MEMBERSHIP IN A GROUP

The second means of gaining some control over the effects of stress is to become part of a group. I suppose there are some few people who are completely self-sufficient, who genuinely feel better outside of a group. A small minority, they are usually more comfortable living alone and show other evidence of really not requiring the presence of other people. But most people need others, and it is vitally important that they establish some sort of regular semi-intimate relationship where they have to come in contact with other people. Outside of the stress of the job and apart from the sometimes difficult intimacy of the family, it is important to have a reason to come together with other humans in a friendly way, buffered by a group.

This human drive has led to the formation of groups of all kinds—religious, fraternal, social, and charitable—and has nurtured their growth. As we have seen, the family is the primary group, the first one that a child comes to recognize, and its support is vital to the healthy individual of any age. The regard the family expresses for its members, the affection that they feel for each other, is important to the individual's social and physical well-being.

But while people should get together with their families, building their ties and strengthening the unit, it is important that each human also relate to groups other than the family. Organizations of all kinds are always actively seeking new members; their welcome is a great ego-builder and they offer most people a supportive relationship that is rewarding and satisfying. Men's and women's service clubs, fellowship organizations, and church-related groups all offer a variety of activities that function as an extended family with the emotional involvements removed. (Although most people come to care very much about their role in the group, it should never approach the emotional complexity of the family.) Most organizations offer a background of people who are interested in you for yourself. It is easy to make friends in the context of a shared interest and most people find fellowship and support within the matrix of an organized group.

Social and service organizations are especially useful for those who need to identify with a cause that is larger than themselves. Political activity seems to provide a good outlet for people who long to be a part of what's going on now. The vast number of activities available assures that everyone who is interested can find a group suited to his needs. Properly used, membership in a group yields sound dividends in two ways: it provides an acceptable escape from the routine of the working life and it establishes without question the genuine worth of the individual.

BASIC HUMAN NEEDS: A SENSE OF SELF-WORTH

This last factor, the establishment of self-esteem and a sense of self-worth, is the third element needed to mediate the effects of stress on the organism. Freudian psychiatry tells us that a sound sense of self is vital to good mental health but, as contemporary man comes to occupy a smaller and smaller part of this complex world, we have begun to realize how important this is to physical well-being as well. There is so much insecurity in present-day living, so much that man is utterly helpless to control, that it is even more vital today that each individual establish a strong sense of self-importance.

As part of a strong family unit most people come to realize at least one aspect of their own importance. People depend on others in the family unit; even the most downtrodden of humans must feel some sense of his worth when he considers his responsibilities to his family. The emotional involvement between parent and child usually develops a strong feeling of importance for both. A parent who has this sort of communicative relationship with his children knows that he is a valuable person to both his spouse and his offspring. This is especially important for someone who receives little in the way of a sense of his own worth from his job.

Other ways of developing a sense of one's importance include accepting positions of responsibility in organizations and the establishment of a hobby. Broadly defined, a hobby is something that you enjoy doing and are willing to work at in a way that develops some expertise. In the normal course a hobby may lead to fellowship with others who share this interest, a valuable and positive form of human contact.

Sports, hobbies, skills, and talents such as painting, sculpture, or music can all be used creatively to develop one's sense of self-worth. Especially later in life, when friends are hard to make and time hangs heavy, it is extremely useful to have developed some type of relaxation that one can rely on to provide both diversion and fellowship. It is enormously satisfying to be a member of a group where one is valued for one's knowledge or background or talent in a shared interest.

Although membership in a group and hobbies appear to be

rather elementary things to do in relation to the prevention of heart disease, it should be emphasized that they provide relief from stress that is extremely beneficial. A strong ego, a sound sense of self, may yet prove one of our most valuable therapies in the struggle against what has been called the atherosclerotic tide.

THE HELPLESSNESS-HOPELESSNESS SYNDROME

Recent work suggests still another way of coping with stress. It appears, although human beings are notoriously unreliable laboratory animals, that the same stress that causes experimental rats to "give up" may also kill humans. The mechanism is not entirely clear but feelings of helplessness and hopelessness seem to precede serious illness with significant, and depressing, frequency.

Internist-psychiatrist Dr. Arthur Schmale carefully plotted emotional states of hospitalized patients prior to the onset of symptoms. His research was careful and objective, and his findings were that most patients had experienced feelings of hopelessness and helplessness immediately preceding their illness. Schmale and his co-workers hypothesize that stress does not *cause* disease but rather seems to promote the conditions that allow disease to appear when it does.

Suggesting that these feelings may set the stage for the appearance of illness, Schmale concludes: "More specifically, this study suggests that the psychic states of helplessness and hopelessness may be related to increased biological vulnerability."

Another psychiatric investigator, Wyler, working some years after the original research, corroborated the earlier findings: "The greater the life change or adaptive requirement, the greater the disruption of bodily function, the greater the vulnerability or lowering of resistance to disease and the more serious the disease that does develop."

At a later medical conference; other investigators reported essentially the same findings. One speaker noted that "up to 80 percent of serious physical illness seems to develop at a time when the victims feel helpless and hopeless."

In practical terms, then, what do these findings mean? Since everyone must face both crisis and stress in the course of a normal lifetime, how can we treat the hopelessness and helplessness that may be the precursor of disease?

From the medical point of view these findings appear to me to present a rather attractive therapeutic possibility. A patient with no history of illness, who is undergoing rather serious strain and who has vague symptoms, obviously needs some supportive counseling in addition to specific medical treatment. Sometimes just talking out his fears and identifying the problem helps; sometimes more direct guidance concerning family interrelationships or career choices is needed. In any case, the presence of overwhelming stress should be suspected whenever symptoms flare up in relation to changes in the patient's life.

It is helpful to direct the patient to more productive ways of handling stress. Although the simplistic advice to "take it easy" is usually worthless, some specific ways of avoiding the feelings of helplessness and hopelessness may be fortifying. For man alone of all the animals has the power, if not to change the circumstances of his environment, then at least to rise above them psychically. People who are made to endure the great stress of imprisonment, for example, discipline their thinking to remain free at least in spirit. And there is evidence that victims who are not overwhelmed by the hopelessness and helplessness of their situation survive, while those who give in often succumb.

The best method of achieving some mastery over a bad situation and one of the keystones of counseling therapy, in fact, is to step back away from the immediate problem and to consider the options available for alternative action. In reality, consciously or otherwise, human beings do this constantly in the course of even an ordinary day: selecting a less crowded street to avoid traffic, choosing to do it the boss's way to avoid an almost certain wrangle, declining to enter a tense situation, carrying enough money to see you through an unforeseen emergency, toting the book you always wanted to read to while away long waits. Each of these provides an alternative to the stress inherent in the situation.

The fuel crisis of 1974 served to bring out the best, and worst, in people. While some sighed and actually experienced depressive symptoms, other people cut wood, rolled newspapers into logs for burning, insulated their homes, and expressed in countless other ways their choice of an alternative to a stressful situation.

Every situation, clearly thought out, reveals a series of alternative actions, an antidote to the feelings of hopelessness and helplessness. When faced with a difficult situation, it is wise to list the possibilities ranging from the clearly unreasonable ("I could run off to Tahiti") to those that on reflection are sound and practical ("I could apologize . . . talk it out . . . borrow money . . . look for another job"). Remember, everyone is down at one time or another; the vast majority are up again in a short time.

Clearly the difference between purposeful behavior in the face of crises and giving in to feelings of hopelessness and helplessness can be the difference between good health and bad.

HOW TO MANAGE THE STRESS OF GRIEF

One of the dismal discoveries of the past decade's research into stress has been the central and significant role of grief. Although folklore has always held that people pine away or die as a result of bereavement, it was not until modern statistical methods were used that we began to realize the enormous destructive power of the stress of grief.

For example, the death rate following the loss of a spouse is *ten times higher* for widows and widowers during the twelve months following the funeral than would be expected, in every age group. In the schedule of recent experiences on page 155, which was developed by asking scores of people to list what they considered the most disruptive events of their lifetime, the death of a spouse consistently ranked first. Divorce is second, both on the schedule and in terms of precipitating disease; the illness rate is twelve times higher than expected in the first year following divorce. The loss of a child has also been documented in the same studies as only the start of a series of events that may include illness, hospitalization, separation, and divorce.

Clearly grief presents perhaps the most acute form of stress that humans must endure; since almost everyone experiences some loss in the course of a lifetime, it is well to know how best to deal with bereavement and loss. The following practical prophylactic measures to understand and cope with these potentially hazardous but almost universal life situations are offered as reasonable means to counter the stress of grief.

First, it should be realized that grief is usually accompanied by physical symptoms that can be dealt with. People who are literally stricken with grief often cannot sleep; they are sometimes unable to eat and find it almost impossible to relax at the time of a death. In some instances the marked stress of the loss of a loved one is related to feelings of guilt or anxiety, the reliving of a lost phenomenon of childhood. At the loss of a parent the surviving children may feel that had they done more, or differently, the parent might not have died. Much of the devastating feeling that follows the loss of a spouse is probably related to unresolved guilt over the marriage relationship itself.

I must point out that each individual must handle these often inappropriate and ill-defined feelings of anxiety as best he can. Often just knowing that such feelings are usual among mourners is enough to get a person through this difficult time. It is also helpful to know that many of the rituals and practices surrounding the event of death are designed to ease these painful anxieties, and I recommend that everyone observe those of his faith to the extent that seems appropriate for him and his family.

The fact that grief is a dangerous and significant stress has been known for centuries and ways of dealing with it have been built into most societies. The ceremonies designed to ease the pain of grief differ in various parts of the world and among various faiths, but in general the traditional means of handling death are ingeniously designed to moderate its effects on the mourners. We may regard some of these practices as primitive or overly demonstrative, but the fact is that observing them helps to expiate some of the residual guilt and anxiety of the bereaved.

Developed with the wisdom of many years, the rituals of grief serve their function well, and I recommend that mourners observe them to the extent that is comfortable for them. No one should feel that because he has not been observant throughout his life he should be denied the comfort of religion and tradition at the time of a loss. The wake ritual in the Catholic faith, the week of profound mourning called shivah observed by Jewish people, and the various other customs in other religions are well worked out and exceedingly valuable supportive therapeutic modalities that should be adhered to as completely as is practicable. Even if they appear excessive they have stood the test of time well and are of great support in alleviating the stress of grief.

It is important that others realize that their role in comforting the bereaved is an important, often health-giving contribution. The visits of friends and family are vital to the eventual recovery of the mourner. Visitors should go out of their way to be supportive, even if the mourner does not appear appreciative or especially social at this time. The value of visits, inherent in the wake or shivah ritual, lies in their impressing the mourner with the fact that other people care enough about him to give their support in spite of his somewhat self-centered disregard of their attention.

In addition to the supportive efforts of friends and family and the observance of the comfort of the rites and rituals of bereavement, there are several other things that can be done to ease the effects of grief. First, it is exceedingly important that the mourner get plenty of sleep. This may be difficult because of the disturbing dreams that may occur somewhat more frequently during the time of mourning, but this just serves to underline the importance of sleep. For it is in the course of sleep disturbed by dreams that many of the unconscious conflicts surrounding death can be worked out. While it is important that the body's physical function be nourished by sleep, it is equally necessary that the psyche be given the opportunity to heal its anxieties at the same time.

The use of sedatives at this time must be judiciously prescribed by a physician whose awareness of the situation is keen and sympathetic. One school of thought holds that it is valuable to shield the individual from the trauma of the first few days by using a sedative or tranquilizer. The other school believes that reaction to death is going to occur anyway, and giving drugs at the beginning when there is still the daily support of friends and family is not the best method of handling grief. If the reality of the situation and the impact of the death hit after the friends and family have reurned to their own pursuits, for some people the stress of grief is increased rather than lessened. Again, this is an individual thing, but as a rule, unless the person is extremely upset, it is probably best to go through most of the early part of the grief reaction with as little pharmacological help as is possible.

For some mourners it is helpful to be allowed to talk: to the noncritical audience of close friends and family it is sometimes therapeutic to ventilate all of one's feelings about the deceased, eulogizing and sanctifying if necessary, in order to rationalize the loss. Good friends will resist the temptation to correct these possibly idealized memories in order to bring the mourner back to reality at this time since it is vital that the mourner express his feelings in whatever way is comforting to him. This idealization of the dead is an important psychological defense mechanism and aids the mourner to adjust to the reality of his life without the loved one over a period of time.

Another physical reaction that can go either of two ways during mourning concerns eating. Some people, suddenly aware of their own mortality, will want to eat voluminously during the mourning period; others will almost completely lose their appetite. It is probably best to allow the mourner to choose his own course, offering food when it is desired and holding back on the comments either way. This is not the time to go on a diet, of course, and since the organism is already stressed by the strain of grief it is probably wise not to indulge in exotic fare.

Sex, and for men the ability to perform, is also affected by the stress of bereavement. (Temporary impotence is often seen following a serious loss of any kind; as I will note later men who are having business problems often experience a short period of sexual inability, the ability to perform either sexually or financially apparently being closely linked in the male psyche.) Other men respond to loss, either personal or financial, by using sex as an escape— sometimes successfully, sometimes not.

Whichever the response, this is a time when a man needs an understanding wife. Although it is true that women's rights in this area are equal to those of men, it is at this point that a loving wife accedes to her husband's needs. If he desires sexual activity she should try to accomodate him; if he does not, this is not the time to berate his temporary sexual inadequacy.

Sexual activity at the time of mourning can be an effective tranquilizing agent for both partners, relieving much of the tension of these difficult days. And if complete satisfaction cannot be achieved at this time by both partners, it should be remembered that affection and physical contact are almost equally important. A severe loss puts a strain on even the most solid marriages; the period of mourning or adjustment should be handled carefully and with control on the part of both husband and wife.

THE SPECIAL DIFFICULTIES OF WIDOWHOOD

The loss of a spouse is perhaps more difficult for a woman than it is for a man. The woman's resources are usually more limited, as is her physical mobility. Very often a widow finds that social opportunities drop off markedly when she is alone. Her life is usually more altered than is a man's in the same situation, the change in her status being much more profound.

Perhaps this is why women frequently fall ill or die suddenly within one year of the death of their husbands. Suddenly alone and usually unprepared, the widow often falls into quite serious emotional depths.

Family, friends, and community can play a major healing role, for it is important that the widow not feel isolated. The cruel phrase, "Let us know if we can do anything," should be instantly replaced by real help in the form of visits, invitations, help with the children, and so on. Even if the widow is not the best company, she should be firmly included in family and social invitations. Insist that she attend, for it is important that she know that she remains a valued friend and member of the community even though she is quite suddenly alone. Friends and family can help by visiting her often, involving her actively in the normal activities of living, and insisting that she participate.

The widow must take herself in hand, and this is easier done when the pressures of friends and family are unremitting. Self-pity and guilt are destructive forces, and she must know that her grief is genuine but limited in time. It is healthful to consider taking a job, getting new interests, and in time finding new male friends. A widow who had been married for some time is like an experienced expert: her talents and abilities will be appreciated by others even if she no longer has a young face or figure.

DEPRESSION FOLLOWING MOURNING

During the period of mourning and shortly thereafter survivors often find that they are depressed. They have little interest in even the routine chores of daily living; their ability to concentrate is impaired and they find themselves unable to either relax or work efficiently.

Be assured that this is a transient and expected thing that almost always occurs following the death of a loved one. With time these mildly distressing reactions fade, and it is important that the mourner understand this. Equally important, he should not immerse himself so totally in the mourning situation that the emotion degenerates into a destructive form of self-pity. This is a negative reaction that can prolong the actual adjustment.

For this reason mourners are advised to surround themselves with other people, first in small groups and then in larger ones. This is often difficult to do and may involve a marked change of habits, especially for those people who had depended heavily on their now-absent spouses. But this is a positive need and friends and family can help immeasurably by trying to get the mourner out of the house and back into the mainstream of living as soon as mourning is completed.

It is also quite normal to expect to grieve quite intensely when alone, giving in at that time to the grief that is never really very far from a bereaved survivor. But moderation in both the extent and length of grieving is important. As time goes on the periods of intense sadness become shorter and shorter and the intervals between them longer and longer. Soon the individual will come to feel that grief has been encountered and controlled; now the time has come to pick up the pieces and to go on living.

Again it is essential to know the difference between a situation one can affect and one which the individual must accept as best he can. The actual circumstance of death is beyond anyone's control. The important thing is that the survivor tell himself that everything was done that could possibly have been done; the mourning has been sincere and heartfelt, the traditions have been observed, and the conflicts resolved. To mourn to the point of illness is destructive; with the help of family and friends and by observing the few rules of common sense set out in this chapter, most people can endure the stress of grief and therefore choose life.

HOW TO MANAGE THE STRESS OF BUSINESS AND FINANCIAL LOSS

At the risk of appearing insensitive I would like to point out that although the death of a loved one is far more devastating than any business or financial loss, the two have many elements in common. Both, of course, create stress situations of considerable magnitude and the difficulties of business reverses are often compounded by extreme feelings of self-hatred and a loss of self-esteem. Because of the destructive effects of these feelings on men of every age, it is vital at the time of business stress that the family work together to bolster the confidence of the breadwinner. The importance of this is underlined by the recent finding that the loss of status and self-esteem is associated to a significant degree with the occurrence of sudden death in men.

I think it is hard for women to understand, but for most men the self-esteem associated with business or professional achievement is of the utmost importance; without it the organism is threatened with a loss that is almost that of life itself. Thus a serious reverse must be handled as the genuine threat it actually is.

It is probably most valuable at this time to emphasize that the individual is not himself responsible for everything that happens to him. Very often a succession of events—most of them beyond his control—determine his success or failure. Rational men should know that most reverses are only temporary and in many cases represent a new and important turning point. Forced to consider alternatives, many men find that what seemed at first to be a catastrophe turns out to be an opportunity. There are countless instances of men who were redirected by events that seemed cataclysmic at the time into new and far more rewarding careers. Every setback should be regarded as no more than a detour—unexpected and sometimes painful but always rewarding in terms of the new opportunity it offers.

But in order to get through the stress of business or financial reverses every man needs two things: an understanding wife and a strong sense of his own self-worth. To be attacked at this time either by a shrewish wife or by serious self-doubt and self-hatred is destructive in the extreme. With the help of a supportive wife, every man can sit back and enumerate his assets. He can honestly say that he is every bit the man he was, strengthened and tempered by difficult times. The stress of a reverse can make a man look creatively at the assets he possesses—in the process often discovering talents that might have lain dormant during normal times.

Destructive ineffective behavior is the real threat at this time. It is too easy to hate yourself, to doubt your worth, especially if your mate chooses this moment to point out your many deficiencies. Sex, too, can be fairly effectively used as a destructive weapon during times of financial reverses. As noted earlier, sexual inability is not uncommon at this time; if either party chooses to use this as an excuse for infidelity or loud argument, it can become a permanent and serious impediment to any kind of worthwhile existence. Like the setback itself, sexual problems at this time are only a temporary disappointment and must not be allowed to become a source of lifelong bitterness.

It is also exceedingly important that the family act to reinforce the father's role. Unless he specifically requests otherwise, every effort should be made to defer to his authority. Although his financial circumstances have changed, it is vital that the man consider himself essential to the family.

An individual enduring the stress of business or financial reverses might do well to remember one fact: once having had success, it is easier to achieve success again. With this confidence and the support of his wife and family, even the most defeated man can regain his "health" in the business and financial world, and maintain physical health as well.

Summary

There are many investigators and physicians (myself included) who feel that stress is the most important coronary risk factor. Since the individual's response to stress determines its effects, the proper attitude can do a great deal to neutralize the damaging properties of emotional stress.

If a person remembers some rather mundane maxims and tries to apply them rigorously, stress *can* be controlled:

1. Also this will pass.
2. It usually is not worth all this aggravation.
3. In six months (or one year, or ten years, or a hundred years) neither I nor anyone else will remember or care about what upsets me so much today.
4. I should not be stressed by those things about which I can do nothing anyway.
5. I must control my responses by responding minimally to minimal stress, moderately to moderate stress, and maximally only to maximal stress. I must learn to recognize which stresses are minimal, moderate, and maximal.
6. Of all assets, the most important is physical and mental well-being.

These are not new, clever, or profound, but they are reasonable, practical, and effective in dealing with stress and thereby the effect of stress on the heart.

Chapter 8

Smoking and How to Stop: Reducing Your Risk of Smoking-Related Illness

Enough has been said about cigarette smoking and its disastrous effects on the health of modern man to render my voice almost unnecessary. No one can be unaware of the dangers of smoking, as experts in numerous medical fields produce study after study proving that smoking greatly increases the risk of illness and death.

Cardiologists, of course, are properly dismayed at the devastating effect of cigarette smoking on the heart and cardiovascular system. Smoking a pack a day increases the potency of any single coronary risk factor at least one-and-a-half times. That is, a forty-five-year-old male, without any other coronary risk factors, whose cholesterol level is 260 mg %, has about one chance in twenty-three of having a heart attack before he is fifty. If he also smokes heavily, his risk rises to about one in thirteen, a staggering demonstration of the additive power of cigarette smoking as a coronary risk factor.

A great deal of statistical work on the epidemiology of cigarette smoking indicates that it is a coronary risk factor with considerable power of its own. In almost every study, cigarette smokers have a greatly increased risk of heart disease; moreover, the risk rises in direct proportion to the amount smoked, heavy smokers having a higher risk of heart disease and sudden death than light ones.

In a large group of patients who were part of the Western Collaborative study the rate of heart attack was 3.6 per 1,000 men per year among those who did not smoke cigarettes; 10.0 per 1,000 men per year in those who did, a threefold increase. Among the smokers the rate was 5.0 per 1,000 per year among those smoking six to fifteen cigarettes a day; and 11.0 per 1,000 men per year in those smoking more than sixteen cigarettes a day.

In a review of twelve years of the Framingham study, reported in 1967, the mortality ratio of smokers to nonsmokers went up with the number of cigarettes smoked per day. In those who smoked zero to thirteen cigarettes per day the ratio to nonsmokers was 90 to 74; in those smoking fourteen to twenty cigarettes it was 121 to 74; of those smoking twenty-one to thirty cigarettes per day it was 159 to 74; and in those smoking over one-and-a-half packs per day the mortality ratio was 169 to 74 or approximately 2.3 to 1.

The effect of cigarette smoking on coronary artery disease is a curious one. Coronary artery disease is ordinarily present symptomatically in three forms: angina, myocardial infarction (heart attack), or sudden death. The correlation between cigarette smoking and the incidence of angina is a poor one; between smoking and myocardial infarction the correlation is more striking but the most significant effect of smoking appears to be its relation to death, especially sudden death, from coronary artery disease. Study after study bears out the findings that fatal heart attacks occur much more frequently among smokers than among noncigarette smokers.

Cigarette smoking also compounds the confusion surrounding the use of other substances. Heavy coffee drinking, for example, is correlated in some studies with increased risk of heart disease; but those who drink a lot of coffee, five cups or more per day, are frequently heavy smokers as well. If smoking habits are considered in the calculation, the association between coffee drinking and coronary artery disease becomes much less meaningful.

Smoking also confuses the relationship of alcohol to coronary artery disease. Heavy alcohol consumers are frequently also heavy cigarette smokers, so it is not clear whether alcohol consumption alone, apart from cigarette smoking, has any effect on coronary artery disease.

In recent studies smoking has been shown to be especially hazardous for women. The data are still coming in, of course, and the cause and effect relationships are still far from conclusive, but as women smoke more they seem to be asserting their right to the same amount of death, disability, and illness experienced by men.

Cardiologists are concerned, for example, because sudden cardiac death, previously almost unknown among women, has now grown to substantial proportions. (The incidence of lung cancer, heretofore a "man's disease," has also risen along with the amount of smoking in women.) Almost all of the women who have died suddenly of cardiac causes have been found to have been heavy smokers, and the role of smoking seems more important in women than it is in men.

In Dr. David Spain's study of sudden death, the grim finding was that in men the ratio of smokers to nonsmokers was 3 to 1; in women the ratio of those who died suddenly was 9 to 1, smokers to nonsmokers, impressive evidence of the increased danger to women of smoking. In the same study the average age of women who were heavy smokers who died suddenly of heart disease was forty-eight years old; nonsmoking women dying suddenly of heart-related causes were about sixty-seven years old, a difference of almost nineteen years. The results of these and other studies demonstrate fairly conclusively that women who smoke wipe out much of the advantage they have always enjoyed over men in terms of risk of heart disease and sudden coronary death. Among nonsmokers who die suddenly of heart disease the ratio of men to women is 11 to 1; among heavy smokers the male to female ratio is only 3.5 to 1.

Women appear to be penalized for smoking in other ways as well. The impact of smoking seems especially strong among those who take the contraceptive pill; complications of hypertension and thromboembolism appear more frequently in women smokers, and there is evidence that the contraceptive pill should be used by this group only when repeated careful studies suggest that no underlying disease has developed. Pregnant women who smoke heavily are at much higher risk for miscarriage, stillbirth, and premature delivery. They tend to have smaller babies and there is other evidence of oxygen impairment throughout pregnancy and delivery. And, as if this were not enough, there is even a study that claims women and men who smoke have more of the crow's feet type of wrinkles.

Health professionals in every field warn of the deleterious effects of smoking on almost every part of the human body. Pulmonary specialists tell of increased risk of lung cancer and emphysema. (The respiratory physicians at my own institution tell me that they rarely see a case of emphysema in someone who has never smoked.) Heavy smokers have much higher rates of lip, throat, and mouth cancer than nonsmokers, and serious periodontal disease seems to flourish in the mouth assaulted hundreds of times each day by the irritants contained in cigarette smoke.

The evidence in the literature is vast and growing larger every day. Regardless of the attempts made by the tobacco industry and others, the fact remains that the data indicating that cigarette smoking is extremely hazardous to the health of man are overwhelming.

SMOKING AND HEART DISEASE: WHAT HAPPENS WHEN SMOKING IS DISCONTINUED?

One of the optimistic findings that has emerged from years of research into the effects of smoking on heart disease is that some studies have demonstrated that people who stop smoking, even after many years, reduce their risk of heart attack almost to that of a similar group that has never smoked. Not all investigators have reached the same conclusion: most of the data suggest, though, that stopping smoking at least substantially reduces the risk of heart disease associated with tobacco use almost immediately.

These are extremely hopeful findings that allow us to emphasize that reducing cigarette smoking, even after years of heavy use, will greatly modify the individual's coronary risk. Even among smokers with symptoms of angina, the risk of more serious events drops when they stop the use of cigarettes. This is especially heartening in view of the fact that cigarette smoking ranks with elevated cholesterol and hypertension as one of the "big three" of coronary risk factors.

THE PHYSIOLOGY OF SMOKING, OR WHY DO PEOPLE SMOKE?

The question remains—with all that is known about the role of smoking in a wide range of human disease and with its known force on sudden death and its contribution to illness and disability, why does anyone continue to smoke?

This may be one of the more significant questions of the era, since almost everyone who is hooked on cigarettes would like to know how to stop the habit. Part of the difficulty of giving up smoking is related to the pleasurable effects of inhaling cigarette smoke. The first puff of the day usually produces a "lift," a noticeably heightened shift from sleep to wakefulness. B. H. Friedman, a recidivist smoker and writer, describes it this way: "without cigarettes . . . I never really wake up—not the way I did when I used to smoke that first cigarette of the day as if I were biting into an alarm clock."

The lift is real because it is produced by stimulation of the sympathetic nervous system. Nicotine activates the release of the chemical messengers epinephrine and norepinephrine from the sympathetic nerve endings. For many people this is the "fun" of smoking, although almost every smoker reports that the lift is most pronounced with the first cigarette of the morning and thereafter lasts only through the first two or three puffs of those smoked in the course of the day. This "jolt" produced by the sympathetic nervous response is what most smokers value most highly.

The obverse side of this release is what concerns most physicians, for the same sympathetic nervous system stimulation that gives the "lift" also leads to an immediate rise in blood pressure and a subsequent increase in heart rate. These effects strain the heart to demand more oxygen and in extreme cases can increase the heart's irritability and trigger rhythm disturbances that can lead to sudden death. Catecholamines released from the sympathetic nervous system by smoking also appear to trigger a rise in blood lipid levels, possibly explaining why smokers tend to have higher triglyceride and cholesterol levels than nonsmokers.

Cigarette smoking also seems to increase the tendency of the blood to clot inappropriately. Patients with circulatory problems or a history of emboli or blood clots are well advised to avoid cigarettes religiously. By constricting the vessels and by increasing the tendency of the platelets to clot, smoking can cause serious, often irreversible problems.

That this predisposition to form clots is related to nicotine was recently demonstrated by research conducted at Tufts New England Medical Center. Volunteers who smoked cigarettes made of lettuce leaves showed no increase in platelet "stickiness," while those who smoked one standard filter cigarette exhibited an increased sensitivity of their platelets to stick together, a process that may be the initial event in the formation of a dangerous and inappropriate clot.

The other pleasurable effect of cigarette smoking is a relaxing one. The increase in blood pressure triggers a reflex that involves the vegetative or parasympathetic nervous system. The heart slows down and a general relaxation follows. For this reason the morning cigarette taken in the bathroom often eases elimination and the one following a meal is so pleasant. But, like the rise in blood pressure, this reflex slowing of the heart can be quite hazardous and may in fact increase cardiac irritability and predispose the smoker to possible dangerous arrhythmias.

Although many people say they smoke for the pleasure they derive from it, others use it as a way to handle stress and anxiety. This seemingly perverse finding is possible because smoking is both a stimulant and a relaxant; as both it is extremely hazardous to the cardiovascular system.

CARBON MONOXIDE, SMOKING, AIR POLLUTION, AND HEART DISEASE

The effects of nicotine have been known for many years, and we recognize that a great deal of the sensual pleasure of cigarettes probably derives from their influence on the nervous system. Cigarettes are first a stimulant, then a relaxant; there is no question that people become habituated by the physical gratification they receive, reinforced by each puff, in the course of a smoking day.

In spite of this, however, efforts have been made to create a nicotine-free cigarette, and I suppose that every smoker has tried the brand advertised to be lowest in nicotine. But most smokers complain that low-nicotine cigarettes cause them to increase the number of cigarettes consumed daily, apparently in an attempt to get the amount of nicotine they desire.

In recent years, however, we have learned something more about the hazards of smoking itself, and there is a growing body of documented research suggesting that, although nicotine affects the cardiovascular system in a deleterious way, smoking itself, by way of the carbon monoxide it produces, may play an important role in the deleterious effects of smoking. These findings concerning carbon monoxide are ominous, since the compound produced by smoking is also a component of air pollution caused by industry and automobile exhaust and also because the carbon monoxide produced by other people's cigarettes may present a health hazard to those who do not smoke but only breathe. What is more, the effects are cumulative: people who smoke heavily in areas of high pollution or on days when pollution is denser than usual are often present in hospital emergency wards with symptoms related to shortness of breath, angina, and, in some cases, myocardial infarction. The problem is considerable in terms of environmental and public health.

Carbon monoxide is a colorless, odorless, and tasteless toxic compound produced during the burning of many substances. When people commit suicide by means of automobile exhaust, it is the carbon monoxide that does them in. It performs its lethal work in the bloodstream by binding tightly to the hemoglobin molecules in the red cells, displacing the oxygen normally carried by these cells. In chemical terms, the hemoglobin in the red blood cells is converted into carboxyhemoglobin, a substance which hampers the vital gas exchange that must take place in the lungs and tissues. The presence of carbon monoxide decreases the amount of oxygen delivered to the myocardium, dangerously impairing the function of the heart. The amount of carbon monoxide present in cigarette smoke is at least *one hundred times* the level thought to be safe in the air we breathe.

In people with angina or circulatory problems, this added compromise can have serious cardiac consequences. In a recent study of men with the leg pains of intermittent claudication, Dr. Wilbert Aronow, of the University of California College of Medicine, concluded that even small amounts of carbon monoxide, measured in parts per million in the air, were enough to impair activity and speed the appearance of pain. The pains of intermittent claudication are similar to those of angina pectoris in that both indicate impaired oxygen delivery to an organ (legs or heart) because of atherosclerosis or hardening of the arteries. Dr. Aronow's research has also confirmed an increased risk of angina pectoris resulting from exposure to carbon monoxide caused by heavy traffic and also as a result of smoking cigarettes regardless of their nicotine content.

Another research group calculates that smokers who have 5

percent of their oxygen-carrying cells replaced by carbon monoxide have twenty-one times the incidence of atherosclerotic disease. Even a level of 2 percent has been shown to have consequences for the human heart. These studies suggest that "there may be no threshold for the effect of carbon monoxide exposure on patients with angina pectoris." Dr. John Goldsmith, of the California State Department of Public Health, goes on to warn in an editorial in the prestigious journal, *Annals of Internal Medicine*: "This possibility requires us to reevaluate the importance of carbon monoxide in heart disease, and it has implications for heart disease patients and for all of us who may be exposed to community air pollution."

These findings concerning the effects of even minimal amounts of carbon monoxide in the air have rightly led to the curtailment of smoking in public places. We applaud the government's moves in these directions and hope to see even stricter control on the carbon monoxide fouling of the atmosphere by industrial and automobile wastes as well as by smoking.

Because the deadly effects of carbon monoxide are additive to those of the nicotine found in most cigarettes, it is easy to see why heavy smokers have a greatly increased risk of serious cardiovascular problems. Heavy traffic, for example, with its periods of idling and deceleration, greatly increases the carbon monoxide pollution in the atmosphere. And an individual who uses this time to smoke increases his exposure to carbon monoxide by a factor that may be enough to produce symptoms. All of the facts are not yet in, but we know enough to warn that this is a dangerous combination and that people with a history of heart disease or angina should avoid heavy traffic and polluted air assiduously. And smoking for this group is an extreme hazard that must be avoided completely.

The role of carbon monoxide in heart disease is still under investigation in laboratories all over the world. A finding of great interest links carbon monoxide to the development of atherosclerotic plaque; on the cellular level carbon monoxide seems to increase the permeability of the cells that line the inside of the blood vessels, facilitating the deposit of plaque. It has also been suggested that carbon monoxide may damage this endothelial lining of the vessels to such an extent that platelets are stimulated to aggregate on this surface. The aggregating platelets release a substance that stimulates a movement of muscle cells into the sub-endothelial vessel layer; these muscle cells have been demonstrated to take up lipids from the blood and eventually form the nidus for an atherosclerotic plaque. Added to the higher cholesterol and triglyceride levels usually found in smokers, this may help explain the common association between smoking and coronary heart disease.

Further studies have linked nicotine to carbon monoxide in an effort to account for some of its considerable lethal power. Dr. Poul Astrup, a Norwegian expert on the role of carbon monoxide in public health problems, discussed this interesting linkage: "Nicotine is probably of minor importance in comparison to carbon monoxide for the association between smoking and athero-sclerosis, but it may have a *synergistic* effect on the carbon monoxide-enhanced accumulation of lipids in arterial walls, and it may also be of importance in the occurrence of arrhythmias in smokers with myocardial damage...."

When all of the research is completed, we will know a great deal more about the often fatal interaction of carbon monoxide and nicotine, and of that among cigarette smoking, air pollution, and the function of the human cardiovascular system. In the mean-while, there is the persistent documented evidence that cigarette smokers die more frequently from heart disease than nonsmokers; the heavier the smoking, the higher the risk of coronary problems. And other studies suggest that cigarette smoking is the factor that increases the incidence of sudden death in young people.

The evidence is compelling. Dr. John Goldsmith, a specialist in the problems of public health, states "cigarette smoking makes the greatest proportionate contribution to the deaths of those under sixty years old, doubling the mortality in several studies. If we can substantially reduce this toll of death and associated disability by reducing carbon monoxide exposure, it would be a massive public health achievement."

HOW TO STOP SMOKING

While we know a great deal about why people smoke and what smoking does to their bodies, we still have not successfully zeroed in on how to make them stop. The pleasure that some people derive from smoking, reinforced hundreds of times each day by every puff, becomes, if not physiologically addictive, then most certainly psychologically habituating. The difficulty of giving up this gratification, coupled in many people's minds with the possibility of gaining weight, persuades even those who recognize the dangers of smoking that they are doomed to a life of cigarettes.

Recent studies concerned with the cessation of smoking, however, offer a great deal of hope, even to the recidivist smoker who has tried to stop but failed. First, there is the fact that millions have successfully kicked the cigarette habit. The National Clearinghouse for Smoking and Health estimates that at least 30 million people in this country have stopped smoking, a number that is swelled by another million each year. This is impressive and incontrovertible evidence that people can and do stop smoking successfully.

Second, help is available today to those who want to stop. There are hospital clinics, private agencies, and smoking therapists, many of which were unknown a decade ago. Depending on your pocketbook, your neighborhood, and your desires, you can obtain practical, effective aid in the struggle to give up smoking. If you are uncertain about the facilities in your area, you might check with the local heart association or cancer society. They often know of agency-supported programs that you can utilize at very little cost.

And there is no shame in trying several of these avenues of escape, for what we do know about the physiology of smoking strongly suggests that there is no one way that works for everybody. (Recognizing this, many of the private clinics offer a return program, free of charge, to any client who is not successful the first time.) The usual pattern of smoking cessation is a rocky one—often several attempts must be made—but the goal is vital and there is no question that even the heaviest smoker can attain it. Smokers who have tried to stop and have failed should be encouraged by the fact that most successful "quitters" have at least one failure in their past.

There are a number of methods that can be used to stop cigarette smoking. These range from stopping cold, to limiting intake, to switching, and finally to a number of techniques that are used by the various clinics for smoking control. (There are also pharmacological methods—using drugs—but these are not usually successful, may possibly be dangerous, and will not be discussed further here.)

Whatever method is used, weight frequently increases when smoking is stopped. Whether this is due to the decrease in nervous stimulation produced by smoking or to the fact that newly stopped smokers replace the oral gratification of cigarettes with candy, chewing gum, and snack foods or whether food just tastes better when cigarettes are abandoned, the reasons are not entirely clear. In any event, it is wise to consider starting a diet at the same time you give up smoking. This can do great things for the ego: attacking and controlling two habits destructive to a person's health cannot help but demonstrate that you have an admirable amount of self-control.

STOPPING COLD

Depending on the individual, this method is either the easiest or the most difficult. If you want to stop cold, the best way is to stop *now*. Not after the next cigarette, or tomorrow, or next week —but right now! Get rid of all the cigarettes that you have in the house and all that you have at work. Do not put away a cache that you plan to use only in emergencies. Throw away every one of the cigarettes in your pocket. Most important, do not announce that you have stopped smoking. People will only laugh or may try to tempt you into smoking again by offering you cigarettes. (Actually, the worst offenders in this regard are often people who have tried to quit themselves and failed.) No matter how much you think you want or deserve a cigarette, do not take one. After two to five days, your craving will wear off and you will begin not to miss it.

You must be serious in your resolve to quit smoking. It is difficult but not impossible. If you do not have the will power for this fairly rigorous cold turkey method, one of the other methods below might work better for you.

(Of marked interest is the striking ease with which smokers of long standing are able to break the habit after they have suffered a heart attack or developed the symptoms of angina. Frequently a frightening event such as this is enough to mobilize the will power—will power that had always been there—to effect the necessary withdrawal from cigarettes. Although this may appear to be locking the barn after the horse has been stolen, even after a heart attack or development of angina, discontinuation of cigarettes can have a significant effect on longevity or on the development of a subsequent problem and is thus a very worthwhile endeavor.)

CUTTING DOWN

The second proven method of stopping smoking is to cut down on the amount of smoking you do. Data from a number of sources demonstrate that the number of cigarettes smoked per day roughly correlates in a linear fashion to the amount of coronary risk related to cigarettes. There are a number of fairly painless ways to cut down.

The first and easiest is to take a pack of cigarettes, dump them out on a table and with a ruler and felt-tip pen mark each cigarette with a circle exactly one inch from its tip. As you smoke the cigarette note the relation of the burning end to the circle and, when the ash reaches any part of the circle, take the cigarette out of your mouth, break it, and throw it away. In this way you will still be getting the gratification of the first few puffs, which are the most enjoyable, and at the same time will be cutting down on the amount that you smoke. (An added dividend to this method is that you will also be markedly cutting down on the tars that you take in. These substances, which may be related to the cancer-producing effects of cigarettes, are in higher concentration in the smoke inhaled from the end of the cigarette than in the part of the cigarette smoked first.)

After a few weeks of smoking only one inch of your cigarette, make the circle three-quarters of an inch from the lighted end; then after a few weeks, make it half an inch, than a quarter of an inch, and finally smoke only one or two puffs. After a week or two of this you will find yourself able to stop entirely.

The second method for cutting down on cigarette consumption is to decide that there are places where you will avoid smoking altogether. Begin with the car, since there is strong evidence that smoking combined with the carbon monoxide of automobile exhaust is an especially hazardous combination. By never smoking in the car you will introduce limited, but fairly regular, nonsmoking periods into your life. And do not let anyone else smoke in your car either.

Then try cutting down on the cigarettes you smoke at work, first at your desk, then during coffee breaks. Smoking at home and at meals can then be reduced until finally there is no place that you will smoke and you will have to quit altogether. Except for the car, the order of cutting down places is up to the individual and can vary, but once you have determined not to smoke in a place, do not change your mind. If you must smoke, leave the place in which you have already decided not to smoke, but never change a designated nonsmoking sanctuary into a smoking place.

A corollary of this method and one that is of value for all who are trying to cut down on smoking is to assiduously obey the law and the no smoking signs. There are many places where smoking is prohibited but where many can be seen smoking. Do not be one of the rule breakers.

The third method for cutting down is to use the clock. Set times for yourself when you can smoke and when you cannot. Thus you may begin by resolving not to smoke before noon or after 10 o'clock at night. When you see that you can control your habit to this extent, increase the time when you cannot smoke—not before 2 o'clock in the afternoon or after 8 o'clock in the evening. Whatever times you set for yourself make sure that you follow your own rules. The demonstration of self-control (and it's not as hard as it sounds) will make extending the nonsmoking times relatively easy.

Another method that is useful is to pick a day or two of the week when you will not smoke. Start with one day during the weeekend and one day during the week. Gradually increase your cigarette-free days until they are every other day; then two of every three days and so on until you are smoking only one or two days a week and then stop. If you use this method it is easier if you start your twenty-four hours of not smoking with sundown and carry it to the next sundown. It is easiest to stop in the evening and the next day to realize that with the coming of darkness you will again be free to smoke a bit, having something to look forward to.

The next method for cutting down is to plan ahead. Decide when you enjoy your cigarettes the most and write down when you will smoke. Your list may include one cigarette after breakfast, one during a coffee break at midmorning, one after lunch, one at mid-afternoon, and one after work. In the evening you may want one after dinner and maybe one while relaxing with the paper or while watching television. You might want to add another cigarette if you plan a stressful activity or for relaxation after it is finished. Add up the number of cigarettes you plan to smoke and carry only that many with you; you will find that in this way you will cut down markedly on the amount of cigarettes that you smoke, especially if you are a heavy smoker.

After a time gradually decrease the number of occasions on which you will allow yourself a cigarette and eventually you will find that you are able to stop altogether.

A similar method is to decide that you will allow yourself only a certain number of cigarettes each day and carry only that many with you. Whenever you feel like smoking, you must realize that if you have that cigarette you will not be able to have one later, in this way learning to conserve your smoking occasions. Also, whenever you finish smoking get rid of the butt so there will be no temptation to relight a burnt-out cigarette when you eventually run out.

All of these methods of cutting down on cigarette consumption can be combined. That is, you may find that circling your cigarettes can be done at the same time you are cutting down on the occasions when you will smoke. Or restricting your daily cigarette intake can be combined with cutting out smoking altogether one or two days a week. Regardless of the method, or methods that you use, be certain that you explicitly follow the rules that you set for yourself. It is imperative that you establish self-control and self-mastery: without these attributes and a strong will to stop, no matter which gimmick you use, you will not succeed.

SWITCHING

One of the most interesting aspects of the relationship between smoking and coronary artery disease is the repeatedly demonstrated epidemiological finding that, although cigarette smokers have a highly significant increase in their risk of heart disease, people who have never smoked cigarettes but who smoke cigars or pipes have about the same risk as nonsmokers.

The reason for this is far from clear. It may have some relation to the manner in which the smoke is absorbed into the body. Cigarette smokers usually inhale the smoke from their cigarettes. The smoke comes in contact with the walls of the thin air sacs deep within the lung. It is here that the air we breathe is separated from the bloodstream by only two layers of cells, the cells of the wall of the capillary that carries the blood and the cells of the wall of the air sac.

In the same way that oxygen passes across these layers of cells into the blood as we breathe, gaseous products of cigarette smoke, including the nicotine, the carbon monoxide, and other substances, pass from the air in the sac into the bloodstream. This exchange occurs rapidly and accounts for the sudden jolt experienced with smoking the first cigarette of the day.

The smoke of cigars and pipe tobacco is also absorbed into the bloodstream but via a different route. Cigar and pipe smoke is too strong to be inhaled and instead the nicotine and other substances are absorbed through the wet membranes of the inside of the mouth. (This absorption route is also used medically for administering nitroglycerin, the small tablets are dissolved under the tongue and the drug is absorbed through the mucous membrane.) This route is somewhat slower than across the air sacs of the lungs and probably less of the carbon monoxide and other substances that may be toxic are absorbed in this way.

Regardless of the mechanism, the low risk associated with smoking a pipe or cigars can be used to advantage by those smokers who find it hard to give up cigarettes. By switching to smoking cigars or a pipe you can avoid the damaging effects on the heart inherent in cigarette smoking.

HOW DOES A CIGARETTE SMOKER SUCCESSFULLY SWITCH TO CIGARS OR A PIPE?

Let us first consider cigars. One of the difficulties usually experienced by cigarette smokers in the switch is that cigars are usually much bigger than a cigarette and last much longer. A cigarette smoker usually wants only five to six minutes of oral gratification; with a cigar he may be stuck with thirty to sixty minutes before it is finished. One of the ways to get around this is to carry a small penknife or cigar scissors; when the smoker has had as much of the cigar as he wishes, he just snips off the burning tip and returns the cigar to his pocket, relighting the cigar later when he again needs a short smoke.

Another problem encountered by cigarette smokers is related to the fact that a cigar usually has a soft end which is clamped between the teeth. This yields more of a tobacco taste in the mouth than most cigarette smokers enjoy, although it is usually highly prized by the confirmed cigar smoker. There are many cigar holders on the market that do away with this problem and I strongly suggest that the cigarette smoker invest in one of them before he attempts the switch to cigars.

It is also wise to embark on cigar smoking with expensive cigars. They smoke easier, taste better, and will make the switch easier and more pleasant. There are many domestic or South American brands that are enjoyable, usually milder than European-type cigars. The small cigars tend to be cheaper but usually contain tobacco of a lesser quality. Often less pleasant to smoke, they are generally not suggested.

Switching to a pipe can be somewhat more difficult and requires an initial investment of both time and money. It is wise to start with an expensive pipe, the more costly pipes being better balanced, lighter, and more comfortable in the mouth. They also smoke cooler, remain lit longer, and are easier to smoke and to clean. It is also important to select the proper pipe tobacco. Here, paradoxically, it is wisest to select an inexpensive tobacco. Newly converted pipe smokers often complain of irritation to the tongue caused by pipe tobacco. This is especially keen when the smoker eats or drinks something acid or carbonated. (Citrus fruit juice and soda especially seem to trigger this irritation.)

Tongue irritation is caused by aromatic tobaccos, the imported ones that smell the best to everyone but the smoker. Tobacco from the southern United States is of the best quality, and in this country is usually the mildest and least expensive. When pipe smoking is first begun it is important that the mildest, least aromatic tobacco be used. Even so, it is helpful to experiment with various brands of pipe tobacco before settling on one type.

Another problem often encountered by the new pipe smoker is related to the increased saliva flow. Much of this saliva finds its way into the stem of the pipe and can be countered by cleaning the pipe frequently both before and after the pipe is used. After each period of smoking is finished, tap out the ash, leaving the small plug of unburned tobacco in the bottom of the bowl of the pipe. Keep your pipe with the bowl part down between smokes; in this way any moisture left in the pipe will drip into the tobacco plug. Just before lighting up again, remove the tobacco plug and run a cleaner through the stem. In this way the pipe will remain clean and much sweeter smoking.

It is also important to learn to smoke a pipe properly. Unlike cigarettes, which are smoked rapidly with frequent puffs, a pipe must be smoked slowly. Feel the bowl of the pipe frequently as you smoke. If the outside of the bowl gets hot, you are smoking too rapidly and may irritate your tongue. A pipe should be puffed often enough so that it stays lit but slowly enough so that the bottom of the bowl remains cool.

Switching to a pipe or cigars is not easy and may take a few weeks to accomplish successfully. With persistence, however, any cigarette smoker can make the switch. The same pleasure received from cigarettes can be obtained from these modes of tobacco smoking without the coronary risk inherent in cigarette smoking.

BEHAVIOR MODIFICATION

Some smoking clinics report considerable success in using the principles of behavior modification, a relatively new addition to the psychological lexicon derived from the behaviorist school. Behavior modification considers the act itself to be the problem—smoking, overweight, or fear of heights—and seeks to alter it. This differs from traditional psychoanalytic theory which seeks the underlying cause. Thus, regardless of whether you smoke because you were weaned too early or crave oral gratification for some other deep-seated unconscious reason, behavior modification offers a method that works by altering the cues that trigger smoking and the pleasure associated with it. Behavior modification attempts lifelong changes in habits, rather than a crash program that may produce only a short-term result.

Proponents of this method suggest that will power has little to do with its successful outcome. Behavior modification aims to change the attitude of the smoker toward the habit so that he can stop smoking and does not even want to smoke. One of the goals of this method is to teach the smoker to respond to the cues that usually trigger smoking—the end of a meal, a television commercial, or the approach of a stressful situation—with activities that replace smoking.

Another aspect of this method involves negative reinforcement, associating smoking with some unpleasant thought such as a vivid picture of death by cancer or the severe chest pains of a heart attack or the constant breathlessness of emphysema. Such negative thinking, if strongly considered and pictured, will take the pleasure from smoking. By then quickly seizing on an alternative activity—an after-dinner walk, sugar-free gum—and by then ending the sequence with the rewarding thought of a cigarette-free existence, people who want to quit are aided in modifying their behavior toward the discontinuance of cigarettes.

This method involves a lot of self-persuasion and borders on gimmickry, but it is effective for many people.

SUCCESS IN QUITTING

The most important element in the conquest of smoking is the individual's confidence in his ultimate success. People with fairly high self-esteem—people who expect to succeed—are usually able to kick the habit. And many report an enormous "lift" from kicking the smoking habit; in control of their destiny, successful nonsmokers are gratified by their ability to live without a crutch they know to be hazardous.

Even those who reported symptoms on quitting—anger, irritation, or depression—expressed their satisfaction on the relatively limited period of these effects (usually only a day or two) and then most emphatically on their ability to live through it, to successfully conquer what had become a serious problem. It is important that smokers who fail, even repeatedly, be assured of their eventual success in the antismoking game. Belief in their ability to prevail is common to all successful nonsmokers, even through one or more tries.

Chapter 9

Overweight
and How to Reduce It:
Rational Dieting

If you are reading this in the subway, at the beach, or in any other public place, just raise your eyes for a moment and look around. Unless you are in a very unusual setting the chances are that most of the people around you, perhaps including you, are overweight. In the United States, most adults weigh at least 5 percent more than their ideal weight, according to tables generated by insurance companies and corroborated by national health surveys.

The presence in our population of this large number of overweight individuals makes us a very fat nation indeed. Obesity, defined as body weight more than 15 percent above normal, is now recognized as one of the country's major health problems. It is associated with increased risk of heart disease and plays a role in the complex patterns of diabetes and high blood pressure.

Obesity also plays an important role in the worldwide epidemiology of heart disease. In parts of the world where food is not abundant and where animal protein is either scarce or costly, few adults are overweight. It is a fact well worth pondering that the rate of heart disease in these so-called "poor" countries is significantly lower than ours. Although life is hard in these protein-poor areas, their male life expectancy is not that much shorter than the well-fed American's.

In terms of heart disease there is little doubt that obesity is associated with greatly increased coronary risks. In the Framingham studies, men who were 20 percent above their ideal weight had an incidence of sudden death that was approximately *three* times that of their leaner contemporaries. This overweight group also developed angina almost twice as frequently as men of normal weight. Other related conditions also appeared more often in heavy men and women than in thin ones.

Obese individuals of both sexes tend to have a higher incidence of hypertension and higher cholesterol levels, two factors that in themselves increase the risk of cardiovascular disease and premature or sudden death. People who are ten to twenty pounds heavier than their ideal weight have a death rate from all causes that is 150 percent that of their less hefty contemporaries.

OBESITY-RELATED HEALTH PROBLEMS

It is easy to understand the reason for this increased incidence of cardiovascular and related troubles. Nutritionists estimate that every excess pound carried on a human frame requires an additional mile of blood vessels; that is, delivering fuel and oxygen to this extra pound of fat cells requires an additional one thousand seven hundred yards of vascular system. Total blood flow must be increased to service these cells and proportionately more cardiac work is required to pump the blood. The hazards of placing this extra burden on a heart already damaged by an infarct should be apparent. One of the clear-cut rules of cardiologic management is that heart attack victims should *always* strive for an optimum weight and should *never* allow themselves to gain more than five or six pounds over their ideal weight. Remember, an extra five pounds of body weight represents almost five miles more work to a heart whose pumping function may already be somewhat impaired.

And the presence of the excess weight itself requires that the body work much harder than it would otherwise. When a man who normally weighs 150 pounds gains an additional 30 pounds, a number of strains are placed on his body. In addition to having to supply blood to the vessels contained in this extra thirty pounds of fat, the heart must also supply the extra blood needed by the muscles to carry around this excess weight. It is exactly the same as strapping a thirty-pound load to the man's back: patients who would not dream of carrying heavy luggage have no qualms about putting on an equivalent amount of weight.

Because fat people must work harder to achieve movement, they usually exercise less and move around less than thin ones. When they must do something requiring effort fat people tend to work up an appetite, because the work they do is so much more strenuous than it would be for those who are not grossly overweight. And so the cycle of less work and more food is embarked upon, usually for a struggle that can last a lifetime.

For these and other reasons, most physicians work seriously with heart patients to simply take the load off. An older physician, a man for whom I have a great deal of respect, told me that he was able to lose weight successfully and permanently when he realized that almost no one he knew over the age of seventy was overweight. Granted that there are exceptions, thin people in general tend to live longer, healthier lives than fat ones.

DIABETES AND OVERWEIGHT

Fat people have a tendency toward diabetes which can develop into clinical, overt disease. In addition to the diabetic symptoms caused by the sparing of sugar—excessive eating and urination, and the elevation of blood sugar itself (usually higher in obese people than in thin ones)—the presence of the diabetic state significantly effects and accelerates the development of atherosclerosis. The mechanism is not clear, but patients with diabetes clearly have a higher incidence of the premature development of heart disease according to statistical measures.

It is interesting that some overt diabetes seen in obese patients disappears when weight is lost. (The management of the disease in those who are overweight almost always begins with stern instructions for weight reduction and a detailed diet.) This "cure" is probably related to the fact that the cells of obese people are relatively nonresponsive to insulin. Although the insulin produced by the body may be adequate, or sometimes even higher than would be needed by a person of normal body weight, the cells of the fat body respond sluggishly to this endogenous, or internally produced, insulin.

In the very obese, insulin resistance of this kind may lead only to mild diabetes, detectable only by sophisticated blood tests. But many patients, even with only moderate obesity, develop the overt symptomatic form of the disease that requires treatment. This insulin resistance is usually not severe and in most cases the diabetes can be treated with weight loss alone or with small drug doses. Even when the symptoms are minimal, however, diabetes has effects on the cardiovascular system.

Obesity also compounds the difficulties and dangers of high blood pressure. Patients who are hypertensive when they are overweight often find that their blood pressure levels return to normal when they lose weight. And the overeating that causes obesity also goes along with an increase in blood lipid levels (cholesterol and triglycerides) that in themselves are associated with coronary artery disease. Reduction of weight will frequently normalize the lipid patterns, especially while the weight is in the process of being lost.

Abnormal triglyceride levels tend to come down dramatically, especially when a diet that is low in carbohydrates is used to reduce the weight. When the weight stabilizes some people remain at the lower levels of blood cholesterol and triglycerides, while others may return to somewhat higher levels requiring further treatment—a specific alteration in their diet or occasionally by the use of lipid-lowering drugs (see Chapter 6).

A WORD ON MODERATION

Now, having said all this and having established myself as antiobesity for the variety of reasons noted, I would now like to affirm my equally strong feeling against the other extreme. Excessive leanness, the kind that is achieved only by what I consider an abnormal preoccupation with self and with dieting, is not desirable either.

Women especially attain the emaciated look favored by high-style magazines only at a very high cost. I have seen too many fashionable women whose size six figures were paid for in terms of irritability, fatigue, tension, depression and, in some cases, even with the loss of their secondary sexual characteristics. (Most women have had the experience of losing their bosom first in the course of an overly strenuous diet.) Nothing is more discouraging to the males who genuinely appreciate women than finding a slim female figure topped by the haggard, wrinkled face of the life-long diet zealot.

Men are rarely as compulsive or destructive in their dieting as women. More often though, failing in their attempt to achieve instant Gary Cooper-type leanness, men will lose patience with the whole diet rationale. Indifference quickly follows—the deadli-est enemy of any diet being the phrase "What the hell?"—and an-other unsuccessful male joins the ranks of permanently fat men.

WHAT SHOULD YOU WEIGH?

Thus standing firmly against obesity, but just as firmly against neurotic overdieting, I suggest that rational adults over the age of thirty-five strive to keep their weight within 10 percent of the ideal given in most insurance tables. This means that a man whose ideal weight is given as 150 pounds should never allow himself to gain, or lose, more than fifteen pounds. His ideal weight, correlated with his height and body build, is somewhere between 135 and 165 pounds. In women I suspect that the range is narrower, perhaps in the area of 5 percent. Thus a 130-pound woman risks wrinkles and a cranky disposition when she struggles to go below 124 pounds; she flirts with fat at 136 pounds and above.

The easiest thing for a physician to say to a patient is "Lose weight." (The second easiest is "Stop smoking.") Neither of these things is easy to do. They are exceedingly difficult and anyone, physician or patient alike, who thinks otherwise either has never tried or is one of those rare people who can control difficult habits like these at will.

For those countless other people who struggle to lose weight or to attain a tobacco-free existence, we will supply rational and effective information—advice that works. It is neither reasonable nor fair for any physician to tell a patient that there is no excuse for not losing weight, to just go ahead and do it. The fact of the matter is that it is difficult but, with sufficient push from the inside and sound advice from the outside, almost everyone can be helped to lose weight.

WHAT DOES NOT WORK: DRUGS

First a word about the drugs that are sometimes used to help patients lose weight. The types of drugs that are used have the effect of either accelerating the metabolism—making the body consume more fuel because it is working harder as a result of the drug's stimulation—or of decreasing the appetite by means of an *anorexiant* effect. Some of the drugs used in the past for dieting contained both anorectics to decrease the appetite and stimulants to increase the rate of consumption of fuel. These drugs were usually of the amphetamine type and included methamphetamine or "speed" and dexedrine, either alone or in combination with a sedative such as a barbiturate or tranquilizer. These were sometimes given alone, with the sedative taken at bedtime, or were combined in one pill.

These are extremely hazardous drugs; I do not recommend or even countenance them for the loss of weight, especially among rational people whose ultimate goal is to avoid heart disease. The effect of these pills is similar to the profound sympathetic nervous system effects discussed earlier. Like a jolt of adrenalin, they increase the heart rate, elevate the blood pressure (sometimes to dangerously high levels), increase the strength of contraction of the heart, and may potentiate blood clotting. As they increase the work of the heart, they also produce agitation and nervousness. The user moves around constantly, thus causing the heart to work even harder.

The speedup of metabolic activity associated with the use of these drugs also produces premature aging in certain individuals, a concept that is difficult to prove but apparent on the faces of lifelong amphetamine addicts. If even minimal coronary atherosclerosis is present, the increase in cardiac work and cardiac oxygen consumption caused by amphetamine-type drugs can also produce the symptoms of angina pectoris and may precipitate a heart attack or serious arrhythmia.

From what is known about "diet" drugs and their effects, I can state most emphatically that they are not safe to use in the fight to lose weight, especially if the goal is to avoid heart disease.

THYROID MEDICATION

Another class of drugs sometimes used in the treatment of overweight is the thyroid hormone group. People with normal thyroid function become mildly hyperthyroid when oral thyroid extract is administered. And hyperthyroid people are usually slender, overweight not being one of their problems. A drawback to this treatment is that the amount of thyroid hormone administered from the outside is not additive to the amount produced by the body. Instead, these drugs inhibit the body's production of thyroid hormone and in essence shut off the gland. To achieve a state of hyperthyroidism, larger doses than are normally produced by the thyroid gland are then needed.

Thyroid extract administered to people whose own glands have been surgically removed or are malfunctioning is a valuable and useful form of therapy. When overseen by a physician, the hypothyroid patient is almost always benefited by exogenously administered thyroid hormone. I am warning here of the use of thyroid hormone given to euthyroid people with normally functioning glands in order to "speed up" the metabolism with the sole purpose of losing weight.

Thus when patients who have been on thyroid drugs for a long time stop their oral medication, there may be a lag until normal thyroid function resumes. These patients may have a period of weakness and lethargy because they are relatively hypothyroid until their own gland resumes its normal function.

Important in the consideration of cardiovascular problems is the fact that thyroid hormone in the dosage used for weight control stimulates the heart to a significant degree. The effects are similar to those of sympathetic stimulation: rapid heart rate (tachycardia) and increased strength of contraction of the heart, two things that increase the work of the heart and the amount of oxygen it needs. There will be an increase in cardiac output that is related to an increase in the rate of the body's metabolism and to the increased production of a large amount of body heat that must be dissipated. When excess thyroid hormone stimulates the heart and increases its need for oxygen, angina or heart attack may occur in people with underlying coronary artery disease.

Thyroid hormone has been found to be beneficial in lowering the cholesterol levels in some types of hyperlipidemias. It has been known for years that patients with hyperthyroidism tend to have lower levels of cholesterol; hypothyroid patients, with poorly functioning glands, tend to have high levels of cholesterol. A form of the drug with reduced metabolic effect, called D-thyroxine, was included in the original design of the Coronary Drug Project because of its cholesterol-lowering effects. Even this less potent form of thyroid hormone had to be discontinued, however, when some arrhythmias were noted in patients on the drug. This less active form of thyroid hormone is still used in the treatment of some forms of elevated cholesterol levels, but its use in patients with heart disease or in those who have already had heart attacks is considered by many to be contraindicated.

The use of thyroid extracts or hormones in the treatment of obese adults with normally functioning glands carries a certain danger with it. The hypermetabolic effects of thyroid hormones along with their increased demands on the capacity of the heart can lead to angina; their continued use can so depress the normal function of the thyroid gland that it may cease to function for uncomfortable periods of time. Although thyroid hormones may lower cholesterol in some people and effect a transient kind of weight loss in others, the artificial induction of hyperthyroidism imposes a dangerous stress on the heart that should be avoided.

"RAINBOW" PILLS

In recent years, until a crackdown by the Food and Drug Administration, various multicolored pills enjoyed a certain vogue among people who were seeking an easy way to lose weight. Dispensed by medical or pseudomedical people, these pills usually were given with instructions to take a yellow one at one time, a green pill later, and still another color at bedtime. Whatever their other qualities, and there is still no evidence that these pills had any but a transient effect on long-term weight loss, these drugs frequently contained digitalis.

Digitalis is a powerful and useful drug, honored by sound medical use over several centuries, that has the effect of increasing the strength of contraction of the heart. Digitalis in its many different forms is the principal drug used for treatment of heart failure and certain rhythm disturbances. It has been said, however, that if Withering were to develop digitalis today, instead of in the seventeenth century when he lived, it could never gain the approval of the Food and Drug Administration. The toxic-therapeutic ratio of digitalis—the amount of drug that will cause toxicity and possibly death as compared to the amount that will yield good therapeutic effect—is much too small to be accepted by the FDA today.

This ratio has been calculated at 2 to 4 to 1: in other words, only two to four times the therapeutic dose may cause serious toxicity and possibly kill the patient. This happens rarely, and under the supervision of a physician the use of digitalis is safe and effective.

But the finding that digitalis in excess of the amount needed to treat heart failure led to a loss of appetite created some reckless interest in its use as an aid to dieting. This *anorexia* or loss of appetite is an early manifestation of digitalis toxicity and rather than an effect to be desired is actually a sign of impending danger. The effects of digitalis toxicity are extremely serious, and include such unpleasant things as nausea and vomiting as well as some potentially dangerous occurrences like atrial and ventricular arrhythmias. The therapeutic uses of this remarkable and effective drug will be discussed in connection with the treatment of heart failure, but it must be emphasized that digitalis, labeled or concealed in the so-called "rainbow pills," should never be used carelessly in the treatment of overweight.

OTHER DIET AIDS

Simple fillers are another type of drug used to treat obesity; these are cellulose nonnutrient foods that are chewed to make the body believe that it is getting something nutritious to eat. What it is getting, in fact, is a form of straw that fills the belly, has no caloric value, and has the effect in some people of taking their minds off food. I would think that making love or a good movie would do a better job of distracting the dieter.

Whether any of the fillers are effective as an aid to dieting is not clear. They are relatively safe compared to the hazards of amphetamines or thyroid extracts or digitalis intoxication. My opinion is that they are probably not effective over the long run. Moreover, chewing these wafers may increase the secretion of stomach acids and enzymes and result in making the dieter feel more hungry. There are no hard data on the subject of fillers but my impression is that they are a fairly ineffective crutch.

We must thus conclude that none of the drugs (other than fillers—which do not work) currently used by some to treat obesity is safe for use in individuals with either overt or latent heart disease. Thyroid extracts and digitalis are safe and effective drugs when used at a physician's direction to treat those conditions for which they are indicated. Amphetamines may also have some limited use in modern medical treatment. But none of these drugs should be "popped" indiscriminately; their effectiveness in weight control is far outweighed by their dangers, especially for the patient with significant or subclinical heart disease.

Moreover, other studies and numerous personal experiences have indicated that none of these drugs is effective for long-term weight control. In almost every case, cessation of the drug is followed almost immediately by weight gain, especially if food habits have not been altered.

It is an inescapable fact: there are only two ways to lose weight. The first is to decrease the amount of fuel available so stored fats will be utilized, a deprivation we call dieting. The other is to increase the requirements for fuel by stepping up the activities of the body, or exercise. As I will note later, properly handled exercise is an effective adjunct to diet in the loss of weight.

WHAT DOES NOT WORK: FAD DIETS

As with everything else in this world, there is a right way and a wrong way to diet. And preeminent among the wrong ways today are the currently popular author-promoted diets.

At the outset, distrust expensive books with titles that promise miracles; invest instead in a pocket-sized calorie counter. Diets labeled Wonder, Miracle, or Revolution and all diets that suggest that calories do not count are inherently dishonest. There are no miracles, only a few shortcuts, and calories do count. About the only thing you will lose in the process of acquiring books of this kind is the $9.95 or so that you must pay for the privilege of owning still another diet tome.

Aside from the misleading titles and dishonest presentation of many of these diet books—unfortunately, only these kinds seem to appeal to the reader while the really sound diet books of the past languish on the shelves someplace—there is evidence that they can do a great deal of harm. Many of the "easy" diet books recommend meals that are high in proteins and drastically lowered, or nonexistent, in carbohydrates. They are effective, at least initially, because this low-carbohydrate diet tends to cause a dramatic loss of water. Fat is not water, however, and this shift in fluid storage produces only a transient loss of some weight, not fat.

More important, people often complain of feeling "lousy" on these expensive high-protein, low-carbohydrate diets, and no wonder. The human brain is engineered to burn nothing but glucose, a high-energy carbohydrate, and our muscles work most efficiently when they are supplied with the same fuel. When starved of carbohydrates the human animal does not work well and usually feels terrible in the bargain.

But the most important drawback to this kind of diet is the composition of the proteins recommended and the high amount of fat that is ingested. The metabolism of protein and fats yields breakdown products in the body that are acidic. This state of acidosis and ketosis has an appetite-lowering effect but also tends to foster a state of malaise. In mid-1973, the Committee on Public Health of the Medical Society of the County of New York took note of the common side effects of diets of this kind: "producing weakness, apathy, dehydration, loss of calcium, nausea, lack of stamina, and a tendency to fainting." The committee denounced that year's fad diet (and its author) as "unscientific . . . unbalanced . . . potentially dangerous."

The fact is that most of the protein available to us is high in fat and high in cholesterol. A diet that stresses both and limits other foods almost entirely can produce chemical imbalances that can lead to kidney disease, heart disease, gout, and other metabolic and systemic problems. If you want to lose weight for the purpose of living the good and healthy life—perhaps reducing the risk of heart disease—then it is manifestly irrational to go on a diet that is high in saturated fats and cholesterol. And since all of the low-carbohydrate, high-protein diets stress foods that are high in fat, their use is extremely unwise. In the presence of underlying conditions of the heart or kidney this extreme chemical imbalance can quite easily precipitate an event that might otherwise never occur.

Diets of the fad type are popular because so many of them are effective in weight loss, for a short time at least. It should be emphasized, however, that the initial weight loss is almost all body fluid, released from the tissues as a result of the carbohydrate deprivation. Another reason for the short-term success of some of the fad diets is the fact that the ingestion of large amounts of fat will in itself decrease the appetite. The animal protein that is allowed without limit on these diets is by nature high in fat, and you can eat just so much of a high-fat meal before you just do not feel like eating any more. If you eat beyond this point, you may become nauseated. Because the fat contained in meat exerts a limiting effect on the appetite, the actual number of calories ingested may go down.

Unfortunately, however, the appetite-cutting effect of high-fat intake is achieved at the cost of dangerous alterations of serum lipid levels and of the body metabolism—often at the cost of a general sense of well-being. Although many of these fad diets or diets that feature a single food are effective for a short period of time, because they cannot possibly be sustained and because they do not alter the individual's eating habits, the lost weight invariably returns, reaccumulating after the diet is stopped.

LIQUID PROTEIN DIETS

Recently there has been much interest among laymen in a technique that has been used by researchers on hospital metabolic wards during the past decade for reducing the weight of massively obese patients (300-600 pounders). The method is essentially fasting with supplementary feeding only of necessary vitamins, minerals and essential amino acids with some protein added. These patients are followed closely with daily testing of blood and urine specimens to ensure that the patient is tolerating this dangerous regimen without serious side effects. Information suggesting that a regimen based on the same principles might be applicable to individuals who are not massively obese, but who have had trouble losing weight on the usual diets, appeared in the mid 1970s and has spurred the development of a new industry producing a liquid protein preparation that its promoters have claimed can be used in place of meals or as the sole intake replacing all food.

Theoretically, the preparation supplies all the necessary proteins including the essential amino acids, which, like vitamins, must be provided in the daily diet. Fats and carbohydrates are not provided, but the body is supposed to be using its own fat stores for fuel rather than breaking down the protein ingested daily or its own muscle for fuel. If it does use its own muscle however, the protein in the diet should replace it. Vitamins and minerals, it has been suggested, should be taken with the supplement, though some brands claim to include the necessary vitamins and minerals. The protein in most of these preparations is derived from the hydrolysis of cowhide, other skins, gelatin and collagen, e.g., gristle.

There are a number of problems associated with the use of this type of regimen. Firstly, when the intake of dietary calories goes down below the amount used in metabolism, almost all of the food ingested, whether carbohydrate, fat or protein, is used as a source of fuel for the body, and the production of muscle is virtually stopped. Moreover, during starvation after the available carbohydrates in the body are used up, muscle that is not constantly in use is used for fuel and last of all fat is utilized. There is no evidence that intake of a small amount of protein will spare the use of muscle for fuel.

It is imperative that this diet regimen be used only under the supervision of a physician. The levels of potassium, sodium, calcium and phosphate in the blood should be carefully monitored and ECGs taken periodically. The potassium level can fall to dangerously low levels even if a supplement is given, because different individuals excrete potassium at different rates. Low levels of potassium in the blood can cause rhythm disturbances in the heart that can lead to sudden death.

An advisory committee to the FDA has recently suggested that this type of dietary regimen not be used by anyone with kidney, liver or cerebrovascular disease; by children, the elderly, or lactating or pregnant women; or by patients who are being treated with diuretics, drugs to lower high blood pressure, oral antidiabetic drugs, insulin, thyroid preparations, or cortisone type drugs. Patients on digitalis should be watched closely for potassium problems.

The side effects noted by this FDA sponsored group included nausea, diarrhea, vomiting, constipation, fainting spells, blackouts, dizziness on changing body position, muscle cramps, heart rhythm disturbances, attacks of gout and nerve damage, in addition to a frequently noted feeling of general bad health. There have been at least ten deaths of otherwise normal individuals associated with the use of these types of supplements in women between twenty-five and forty-four years old. Eight of the women died with intractable ventricular fibrillation (the most ominous heart rhythm disturbance) and could not be resuscitated. Five of them had evidence of heart damage, even though their coronary arteries were normal.

Another potential hazard of these liquid protein diet supplements, in addition to the fact that the protein is frequently of low grade nutritionally and may not provide the necessary amino acids, is that the product is an excellent culture medium for the growth of bacteria. Any contaminated batches or swollen cans should not be used. The material should be refrigerated after the can is opened or the powder is mixed with liquid, and it should be used promptly.

After being on this type of diet for a time, one should return to a normal diet slowly, over two or three weeks; three reported deaths occurred in patients resuming their normal diets.

These diets, though they are frequently effective over the short run, do not change the habits of the dieter, and soon after the usual diet is resumed, weight reaccumulates. Because of the many problems and dangers associated with this diet regimen, it cannot be recommended except in extraordinary situations and only in a hospital setting or under the care of a physician experienced in the management of these diets.

SOME SUCCESSFUL TECHNIQUES

Before we dismiss all popular diets as ineffective or possibly dangerous, a word about the various groups that have been formed throughout the country for the purpose of weight reduction. Most of them follow principles that are at least partially based on the successful operating techniques of Alcoholics Anonymous.

Their supportive methods have proven successful for many people who need help in their struggle to lose weight or to avoid alcohol. It is interesting that just as Alcoholics Anonymous is the one consistently successful method for maintaining former alcoholics, reducing programs modeled after it seem to be most successful over long periods of time in the control of weight problems.

The techniques used emphasize support, with group meetings providing both comradeship and the gratification received from the approval of one's peers. This positive reinforcement enables members of these groups to succeed for long periods in the program. Within the structure of the group, participants who have lost weight in the course of the week relate how they have successfully withstood temptations of all kinds. The dieter receives the instant approval of his fellow weight strugglers, often before any results can be seen in the mirror. If he has not lost weight, the dieter is stimulated to continue in his efforts by the realization that others in the group have been able to overcome exactly the same temptations that have beset him. The weekly weigh-in, whether or not it shows a loss, is effective in the same way that a regular appointment with a physician would be.

The most effective weight control groups also provide diet tips and recipes that are usually quite sound. These seem especially valuable for women who find themselves housebound by young children, often a time of greatest weight gain for new mothers. Unfortunately, women who are home a great deal of the time are constantly exposed to the joys, and risks, of an open kitchen. But the homemaker who really enjoys cooking can spend hours in the kitchen happily preparing foods that are good to eat and remarkably low in calories. By following the recipes distributed by the weight control groups or those contained in some of the sound diet cookbooks, an amazing variety of foods can be prepared to satisfy even the most demanding dieter. I am especially impressed by their ideas for snack-type foods, an area where even the most careful dieter may have trouble.

The rational dieter, however, should approach even these programs warily. Some of their meal plans allow far more eggs than I would like to see, and unless hot dogs are drastically reformulated, I strongly recommend that they be replaced by a fish or fowl meal. Some dieters with sensitive gastrointestinal tracts might also find some of their suggestions too spicy and they are well advised to cut down on the condiments permitted.

While on the general subject of visits to the physician I would like to emphasize that no one should undertake a rigorous weight reduction program of any kind without checking first with his doctor to rule out the presence of any condition that would contraindicate dieting of any kind. Although the diet outlined in this chapter is safe and rational, each individual must be guided by his physician in matters of drastic diet alteration.

Successful Dieting

If drugs carry a considerable risk of taxing the heart to a dangerous extent, and if the well-publicized "easy" diets are irrational because of the high amounts of animal fats they contain, how does one go about losing weight safely and effectively?

Let me first assure the reader that it can be done. I have had many sensible patients whose weight loss has been a factor in their lifelong good health. Considerable weight loss has in some patients controlled the diabetes or high blood pressure that I detected on examination, and in others has reduced previously high levels of blood lipids to limits that are considered safe.

REALISTIC GOAL

In analyzing what distinguishes successful from unsuccessful dieters I am struck by several things. First it seems to me that all the successful dieters I know had decided on a realistic goal. Determining how much weight to lose and how quickly to lose it appear to be prerequisite to success in dieting. The key here though is the word "realistic." Unfortunately, our society appears to have a culturally imposed, esthetic preoccupation with thinness. To be very stylish and "with it" today means to be exceedingly slender. Although many reasons have been advanced for this focus on being thin, it may not be a realistic goal for many people and often leads to frustration and defeat in dieting.

If a mature male, endowed by nature with a short or heavy frame, tries to achieve the unrealistic goal of looking like a thin, perennially young television performer, he is almost always doomed to failure. It is far more realistic for men to try to return to the weight they were when they last considered themselves to be in good shape. Assuming that they were not obese from childhood on, most men are at their optimum body weight around age twenty-five. With marriage, changing interests, decreasing activity, and increases in eating and drinking, corpulence follows. Metabolism slows, less fuel is required, and the excess is stored as fat. In our society, few married men get regular and vigorous exercise. As men become successful and accustomed to affluence, they tend to eat more and better, and to move around less.

I recently scolded a patient for consistently weighing at least thirty pounds more than was good for him. He argued that my office scale had to be wrong—"heavy"—because he was certain that he had not gained more than one pound each year since he was in the army! A little rapid arithmetic proved that even a pound a year adds up to obesity by middle age.

In general men do not have the patience to attain a specific weight or waistline. It is more effective to get down to the weight where you look the way you think you should, where you can go into a store and buy a suit that fits in the shoulders and does not have to be let out in the waist or trousers. Other good tests are the ability to wear regular, rather than portly or outsize sizes, with no need to move jacket buttons to accomodate a frontal corpulence.

Often it is not necessary to lose as many pounds as you think, although there are a number of tables that give a range of ideal weights for men and women. For some individuals it is almost impossible to achieve these "ideal" body weights, especially at more mature ages; they either feel terrible as the diet proceeds or find that maintaining the new lowered weight is just not feasible. Very frequently if the goal is unrealistic the weight stays down for only a short time and then bounces up again. This is extremely discouraging and should be avoided like the plague it is.

The problem of unrealistic goals is even more prevalent among the women in this society who would like to look, unfortunately, like undernourished seventeen-year-olds. If this unrealistic goal is achieved, it is often at the expense of a sense of well-being and good health, and sometimes of beauty itself. Most women blossom between the ages of sixteen and twenty-six and at this age most women do not even have to think about what they eat. With the active metabolism of youth, a woman who can eat a great deal without gaining weight also appears at this age to be able to lose unwanted pounds rather easily.

As most women reach the age of thirty and beyond, their need for calories decreases and they begin to put weight on, just as men do. In limited amounts, it is nature's way of filling out tissues that would otherwise be prematurely aged. If a mature woman does manage to starve herself into a tiny youthful size, it is often at the cost of both health and beauty. Except for very small-boned individuals, it is unrealistic for a woman of forty or older to expect to fit into a size five or six. While overweight is a definite health hazard, prior to the age of menopause it is not clear whether weight loss in women has much effect on the development of atherosclerosis. Strenuous dieting in younger women must therefore be regarded as cosmetic, rather than healthful, in motivation.

Mature women who wish to achieve slenderness and remain unwrinkled would do well to diet moderately, *all the time*. That means to avoid binges of eating as well as periods of starvation. Again the goal should be a certain body image rather than a specific weight or dress size. One of the easiest ways to determine this goal is to apply what I call the face-to-body ratio.

For Women: The Face-to-Body Ratio

A favorable face-to-body ratio insures a relatively unwrinkled face while it allows a relatively young and slender figure. As women mature, their aim should be to exchange the titillating prettiness of youth—which is always lost anyway—for the handsomeness of maturity. If this is to be done with any measure of attractiveness, some fat cells must be present in order to maintain a smooth and unwrinkled visage. There are other elements to aging, of course, sunlight and heredity being two prime ones, but a few added pounds offer some protection against the wrinkles that appear with age. Most important, the rapid or drastic weight loss that could be tolerated at a younger age without loss of skin tone and tightness simply cannot be handled well by women who are past the age of thirty.

As is the case with men, the goal at all times should be to maintain a sensible weight. Women should enter their middle years with a smile, a sense of great adventures to come, and a comfortable weight margin of no more than 5 percent of their ideal weight. The goal at all times should be an appropriate rather than an emaciated figure. A cushion of two or three pounds will keep time on your side in the never-ending struggle to keep the face-to-body ration in favorable balance. A very slim figure attained at the expense of the face almost always results in the wrinkles and premature aging that characterize the diet zealot.

Classic beauty in women has long been associated with the full figure that offers some insurance against the ravages of age. It is only recently that those two destructors of female youth and beauty, the year-round suntan and the very thin body, have been thought to be fashionable. But now the possibility has been raised that the superthin vogue is one possible cause of the greatly increased incidence of depressive illness among women.

In apparently increasing numbers, women of middle age and beyond seem prone to depression, anxiety, irritability, and a whole spectrum of psychosocial complaints. Many reasons have been advanced for this, including menopause and its hormonal changes, but in some cases the terrible dissatisfactions of these women with themselves and their lives can be traced to destructive dieting. Concerned about the passing years, possibly jolted by a nest suddenly empty of children, some women apparently seize upon dieting as the thing to do—and often subject themselves to the strain of chronic hunger and in extreme cases to actual malnourishment.

Hungry, cranky, and dissatisfied women have problems of a complex nature, obviously; depressive illness is an extremely serious condition that can be treated only with difficulty. Women who risk precipitating it by dieting recklessly are extremely ill-advised, both by the magazines they read and the shallow values they seize upon. For reasons of good health, mental and physical, women should make a realistic assessment of their age and body build; they should enter their middle years with the few pounds they need to maintain a favorable face-to-body ratio and they should strive to avoid repeated excessive weight losses and gains.

THE HAZARDS OF GAINING AND LOSING WEIGHT

Dropping considerable weight and then gaining it back again may be possibly worse for your health than having a stable but somewhat elevated weight. This is because each time you lose weight you lose, in addition to the fat, some muscle mass or lean tissue. When you regain the lost weight unfortunately you do not regain the lean tissue; lost pounds that are regained consist almost entirely of fat. The loss of lean tissue may lead to chronic tiredness and many accelerate the appearance of age. Weight-bobbing also has a deleterious effect on the levels of cholesterol and triglycerides in the blood.

PERSONALIZE YOUR DIET

The second element shared by almost all of the successful dieters I know has to do with the selection of the proper diet. While some few people are happy when given a diet sheet that tells them exactly what to eat at each meal, most humans express their individuality by preferring certain foods over others in daily patterns that are not the same for everyone. For long-term weight control I think it is probably more effective to know which foods to avoid and how to handle portion control, two necessary elements of any diet.

You are ahead then if you structure *your* diet around *your* preferences. If you have never eaten breakfast and are comfortable with only two meals a day, then by all means continue in this way. The time when you are trying to lose weight is not the time to add a meal that you have never found necessary. Many people find that they are more hungry all day if they start off with a substantial morning meal; others cannot start the day without a good breakfast. If you are one of the latter, you will have to allot a third, more or less depending on your needs, of your food intake to this meal. If you are one of the former and can get along with little or no breakfast, then you will almost certainly make up for this meal in the course of the day.

Successful dieting requires that you handle these details yourself. Find the pattern of food intake that is most comfortable for you, for you will want to stick with it for the rest of your life—not hysterically or excessively but quietly and steadily toward the goal of good health. Structure your diet around your special needs. If you are absolutely empty and dragging late in the afternoon, try saving your luncheon dessert for then or have some fruit or cheese. If a cocktail before dinner is absolutely essential to your sense of a good life, go easy on some other source of carbohydrate— eliminate a piece of bread for instance—and enjoy your drink. You can probably save considerable calories in this regard if you use a pocket guide to compare the calorie count of various beverages and their sneaky mixers. If you are going to have one or two drinks every evening, then you should use club soda or plain water in place of tonic or ginger ale. The same is true of the alcohol itself. The number of calories per "shot" goes up with the "proof" of the beverage selected, ranging from 46 calories per ounce in sherry to 83 calories in a one-ounce shot of vodka. Use a calorie counter to be sure you are not taking in far more calories than you imagine.

Think for a moment about your pattern of snacking, since this is often the source of a large number of calories that you may not even by aware of. This is where calorie counting is an eye-opener, since that handful of peanuts that you hardly remember taking can add up to a whopping 250 calories. Apple pie will add another

560, while potato chips and pretzels in sufficient amounts can total almost as much as a meal. Evening snacks seem to prove most difficult for most people; other than going to bed early there is not a great deal to do about mindless eating at this time. Try removing yourself physically from the candy dish. Keep the refrigerator filled with low-calorie vegetable snacks, and try dipping them into the low-calorie dip that is suggested by several of the national weight reducing organizations. These "crudities" yield a lot of chewing satisfaction for their few calories and keep your hands busy besides.

If you find that snacks are an important part of your daily intake, you must design your meals around them. Some successful dieters eat nothing but snacks, preferring to take in their daily calorie allotment in the course of six or seven small meals a day. The important thing, of course, is to plan your daily food intake around *your* likes and dislikes and to structure your meals on the schedule you find most congenial.

COUNTING CALORIES

In general a reducing diet is just that: the ingestion of fewer calories than you need in order to force the body to burn the fat stored in its depots. But here again the operative word is "reduce"; you will simply have to eat less than you are accustomed to. With the help of a good calorie counter you can determine exactly how many calories you take in each day. Depending upon your level of activity and the rate at which you burn calories, you will lose weight if you take in 1,200 to 1,400 calories a day. This is a personal matter, of course, and if you wish to cut down moderately and lose weight more slowly set your goal loosely at 1,600 calories a day. The important thing is to eat less, avoid fattening foods altogether except for well-designed cheating, and find a method of doing what is most comfortable for you.

If you really enjoy counting calories be sure to list everything that you have eaten in the course of the day. This is sometimes a good method to use in starting a diet, for it is an eye-opener to discover how many calories are taken in almost unknowingly in the course of a day. Counting calories also has the advantage of allowing you to substitute foods more accurately. If you keep an honest count and enjoy living dangerously, then it is no problem to substitute a hot fudge sundae for half of your daily intake, or 700 calories taken in some other form. The cheating meal, discussed later in this chapter, will also permit you to indulge in this form of madness.

The alternate method of dieting is to cut down or cut out, the object being to limit your intake of fattening foods. This allows you to eat fairly normally and minimizes what you have to remember, a valuable aid sometimes for men who must eat a certain number of meals away from home.

Either way be sure to find the diet that is most congenial for you. Structure it around your likes and dislikes, tailor it to your lifestyle, stick to it honestly, and you are halfway home.

A WORD OF CAUTION

For men and women who have decided on weight goals that are realistic in terms of age and body build and who have taken the time to determine how they want to structure their food intake, a few words on what to expect from this or any other diet. First of all, there is an inertia to weight loss, a tendency for things that are moving to keep moving and for things that are at rest to remain at rest unless considerable extra effort is exerted. This means, unfortunately, that not much weight is lost in the first two or three weeks of dieting. The occasional drop of several pounds at the start of a diet is usually only water and this does not amount to much over the long run. It is sometimes helpful to limit salt intake, especially at the start of a diet regimen. This helps to drain water from the tissues and often produces a gratifying effect at the first several weigh-ins. Reducing carbohydrate intake also helps to flush excess fluid from the body tissues.

But in some people there may be a period of two to three weeks of dieting before there is any significant weight loss. That the reverse is also true—weight loss may continue after strict dieting ends and a week or two of good eating may result in no weight gain—may be one of the reasons that compulsive dieters tend to bob back and forth between high and low weights. They get down to their desired weight at a realistic one to one-and-a-half pounds a week; they stop dieting strenuously and are delighted to find that they continue to lose weight at the same rate for a couple of weeks. By this time they really think they have it made and, throwing caution to the wind, they return happily to the foods they ate before they started to diet.

Since there is no immediate weight gain, the once controlled dieter is off on a binge that may prove destructive. Not realizing that this is the obverse side of the inertia that rules in weight loss, he indulges in the larger diet, even increasing the amount of food eaten as a reward for doing such a good job and losing so much weight.

Sometimes unfortunately dieters can eat like this for as long as a month with no noticeable increase in weight. By the time the pounds have begun to return they are back in the habit of excessive calorie intake and the scale shows the inexorable effects of inertia once again. In a very short time the recidivist dieters are back where they started, often with a few pounds added. The serious dieter should not be disappointed if it takes a while before weight starts to move off the body, and he should not be deluded by the fact that once the weight is down he may be able to continue to lose weight while eating increased amounts of food. In both cases, it is only a matter of time—and inertia.

Do You Sincerely Want to Lose Weight?

Successful dieters know with certainty that they want to lose weight. They have dallied with the thought before and even tried a couple of diets and failed. At some point, however, usually after a good hard look in the mirror, they must decide that they really want to lose weight. At this point a crash diet or a drug-assisted fling is most tempting, for it promises quick and easy results.

But the rational dieter will recall that all drugs used to speed up the metabolism or otherwise help in weight loss are dangerous and irrational; fad diets are no safer, and in any case weight lost in this way returns all too soon. If you really want to lose weight and keep it off, a definite long-term emotional commitment to a certain pattern of eating must be made.

Every doctor has been impressed with how easily a patient can lose weight if he has been frightened by a heart attack, or by the doctor's warning that he risks the rapid development of serious heart trouble if he does not shape up. It is sad to note how quickly a woman can get herself into shape, losing weight rapidly and successfully, if she suddenly finds herself a competitor in the marriage

market. Women who remain obese during their marriage sometimes find that they have the drive to lose weight if they lose their
husbands through death or divorce and suddenly find that they
must compete for jobs and for men in a young and slender world.

For mature people, it is essential that this kind of lifelong
commitment be made in good faith. If a person really does not
care, likes the way he looks and the way he eats, and is genuinely
unconcerned about what his eating habits may be doing to his
chances for a long life and good health, then the haranguing of his
family and his physician will do little good. Each man must decide
for himself that he genuinely wants to lose weight. He must know
that he will probably have to control his eating habits throughout
his life, that he will have to "watch" constantly.

I have often thought that, since there are so few things in life
that we can effect ourselves and so little direct control that we can
exert individually, perhaps dieting should be approached as a
worthwhile personal challenge. A contest perhaps, where hard in-
dividualistic and self-directed effort can pay off in terms of good
health and a marvelous sense of having triumphed over a difficult
opponent.

As a physician I have often noted the genuine satisfaction
radiated by the successful dieter. When he even begins to near his
ideal weight, the successful dieter experiences a sense of well-being
that is truly remarkable. The formerly obese person looks better;
he has more confidence; his general health improves and he is in
every way a successful human being. It is a goal that is well worth
pursuing.

I should mention that the reasons for gaining a great deal of
weight are strangely atavistic. Eons ago, when life was cruel and
uncertain, the animal who could store fat had an increased ability
to survive famine. When food was scarce he could hibernate, reduce his activities to the minimum, and live off the fat stored by
his cells. But in the ordinary course of present-day living we do not
have to cope with conditions of famine; stored fat presents more
of a threat to us than any real shortage of food. The tendency to
store fuel as fat is a negative, rather than a positive, survival factor
today.

A great deal has been written about the emotional components of excess weight: fat laid down as insulation against other

people by those who do not relate well, certain sexual fears of fat people that cause them to make themselves physically unattractive, the need of fat people for love which they take in the form of food, and so on. All of these may be true, and you have my sympathy if you developed a lifelong fondness for chocolate cupcakes because your mother gave them to you as a sign of approval. But I must point out that, although all of these things may operate to some extent in the pathophysiology of obesity, they also constitute an incredibly garbled psychological crutch. When you are grown up and excess body fat makes you unhappy, unattractive, and possibly ill, then it is time to throw away the excuses and leave the tortured jargon to those who really need it. Waste no time worrying that a weight loss may change your body image and produce some risk of psychological maladjustment; except among the very ill, weight loss is almost always a physical and psychic "lift." Earn it and enjoy it.

How to Stick to Your Diet

Begin by not expecting too much too soon. Since you are embarking on a sensible program of nutritious eating, you should not expect to lose more than a pound or two at the most each week. If you are losing more the diet may be too strenuous and impossible to stick to for more than a short period of time. Once weight loss has begun it will continue at this sensible and steady rate as long as you wish it to, and in this way you can maintain the goal you envision.

At the start you may find that you are hungry most of the time. These are truly difficult times, and you can best get through them by keeping busy, visualizing the new slim you, and eating immoderate amounts of calorie-free snacks like celery, mushrooms, and carrot curls. Stock the refrigerator with cold chicken for an occasional late night snack, and drink plenty of club soda, garnished with a slice of lemon, for a cool summertime treat. In the winter fill your belly with low-calorie hot bouillon, clam broth, or lightly sweeetened tea or coffee. If you make an effort to take your mind off food, happily rather than with bitterness, and if you keep busy you will find it easier to get through the first weeks. By limiting salt and losing some fluid, you may show an early weight loss that will help immeasurably to get through these first few days.

At this point it is probably a good idea to increase your physical activity somewhat. A moderate amount of exercise taken *regularly* each day helps considerably by burning calories. It also helps in your struggle to eat less since nothing is more conducive to thoughts of food than inactivity. Try taking a walk each night after dinner; it helps to burn calories while it effectively removes you from the table where the temptation to clean the plates may be strong.

Being somewhat hungry is to be expected, but do not delude yourself into thinking that the presence of hunger is a reliable sign that you are dieting enough. The sensation of hunger is, for many overweight people, not necessarily associated with a lack of calories but can be triggered even after a gluttonous meal by the sight of a tempting dessert. Even unsuccessful dieters, who actually gain weight during a "kidding-themselves" diet, will experience hunger because they are always thinking about food.

CHEATING

One thing that will make it easier to stick to your diet is the cheating that I most strongly recommend. It is a key part of the diet regimen that I have found successful and I suggest it to all my patients. But it is essential that the dieter be completely honest with himself on the subject of cheating; he must know when he is cheating and when he is dieting. Indiscriminate cheating, not knowing the difference or not being honest about it, is the destruction of this or any other kind of dieting.

Limited cheating once a week is vital because it allows you to have a short and relatively insignificant fling without going off your diet. Everyone knows the hideous guilt of dieting successfully for a short period of time and then going on a binge that somehow triggers the response of never again resuming the diet. The mechanism seems to be that falling off the wagon once means the end of dieting, sometimes forever. I would like to see an end to this kind of thinking; it is destructive and inhuman and probably accounts for more lapsed dieters than any other.

What I suggest is that once a week the dieter plan to eat the thing he has missed the most during the week. For many people this makes the week's struggle with food bearable; the dieter looks forward to this meal with an anticipation that is almost sensual in nature. But it is absolutely essential that cheating be done with style and control. If you cheat a little here and a little there, before you know it you are cheating all the time and the diet is done. I recommend that you cheat all at once, really big, and that you limit your cheating to one meal each week. If you go out for dinner with friends this may be the time to cheat; first of all, it's spectacular to dine with a dieter who is eating everything and you may become the envy of the neighborhood; second, it will probably make it easier for you to get through the weekend, always a perilous time for dieting.

But effective cheating requires that the dieter be absolutely honest with himself. He must know when he is dieting and when he is cheating; this requires that you plan the cheating time beforehand and stick to it. It is also essential that the dieter not cheat more than once a week; if you are cheating more often you are not dieting. And the cheating should be done in *types* of food rather than in *amounts*. Do not think of your cheating meal as an enormous excursion into forbidden territory. Once you have accustomed your body to a lowered intake of food, it is senseless to gorge. It is far more effective to go into a good restaurant and order well-prepared foods that are taboo on this or any diet. During your cheating meal you will eat the portion that is served, enjoy it thoroughly, but please do not ask for doubles.

Some of my patients tell me that at their cheating meal they taste *everything* that is not on their diet, not in tremendous amounts because that is not allowed, but they get at least a taste of everything that they have thought about during the week of dieting. I have another patient who goes to the movies once a week, spending at least a dollar and one half on candy and popcorn before he takes his seat. This is actually a very effective cheating meal because you can eat only so much candy and popcorn, even in the dark warmth of a movie theater. Other dieters will have a fairly sensible meat and vegetable meal but top it off with a dessert that is truly spectacular.

In these ways the dieter gets the tastes he has been dreaming about all through the week. As you can see, the amount of food taken in at the cheating meal will not make that much difference over the long-term course of the diet and the serious dieter will be strengthened in his resolve to get through still another week on his rather limited program. Most important, the cheating dieter knows that he will cheat, that he will enjoy it, and that he will go right back on the diet, and stick to it.

WEIGH IN

For some people it may be helpful to see a physician regularly for diet control; others find the weekly meetings of diet groups an effective way of staying within the limits of their goals. For dieters who are doing it on their own, it is necessary to understand the proper use of the bathroom scale. You must know, of course, how you are doing on your diet but this requires that your scale not be overused.

Weigh yourself on the same scale, in the same room, at approximately the same time—but only once a week. Since weight fluctuates widely from day to day, sometimes even in the course of one day, it may be discouraging if you weigh in more often than once a week. Every Friday morning, for instance, after evacuating the bowels and bladder, weigh yourself and record the weight on a pad kept for convenience near the scale; try not to consult the scale again for another week.

Weighing in every day is of little value, and may be especially discouraging to women whose weight seems to vary widely according to where they are in their cycle. Although much of this weight is lost again after the onset of menses, it is terribly discouraging to women dieters to find that they have lost little, or in some cases gained a bit, while on their diet.

Since men's weight varies too, there is not much point in anyone weighing in more frequently than once a week. It is sensible to have the cheating meal sometime after the weight has been taken, never before, because any transient weight gain can be disheartening. With the weight taken only every seventh day, there should be a noticeable drop after the second week. If this does not occur, the diet is too liberal or the dieter is being less than honest about his adherence to it. He should check the actual number of calories he is ingesting and should especially note the sizes of the portions of each food that he is eating.

How to Do It

The diet suggested here is safe for most people. It should not, however, be thought of as a physician-prescribed diet that is safe for everyone. If you have any physical problems such as diabetes, gout, or ulcers—if you have known systemic or organic disorders of any kind—it is important that you see your physician for an individualized weight reduction program that is suitable for your condition. If there is any question, if you have not seen your doctor for a year or more, or if you are planning a severely limited diet, then by all means make an appointment to see your physician without delay. Obtain his approval for this or any other diet.

Any diet that results in a weight loss is going to be reduced in calories. Although it may be chic to write that calories do not count, the truth is that they count for everything. Whether you reduce them sensibly or by some bizarre manipulation of diet, how many calories you take in determines how much weight you will lose.

A pound is equal to about 454 grams; each gram of fat, which is what we are struggling to lose, is the equivalent of 9 calories. Simple arithmetic indicates that to lose one pound of fat we have to either deprive ourselves of 9 times 454, or approximately 4,000 calories, or we have to increase the amount of our activity to the extent that an additional 4,000 calories are burned up. If you choose the diet route, which is sensible because you can augment its effects by increasing your activities somewhat, then in the course of a week you should take in 600 calories less each day than you actually use to achieve the goal of a one-pound weight loss (7 days × 600 calories = 4,200 calories or about one pound of fat) per week.

Most men eat at least 3,500 calories daily, and most women about 3,000. And they are relatively in balance: that is, the activity they do and the food they take in usually are about equal in energy. There is rarely a negative balance because when people burn more than they eat they begin to get hungry and most respond to this signal by eating more.

Reducing your intake of calories is a highly personal matter and should be done in a way that allows for your preferences for

specific foods. There are many good calorie counters on the market
—the most useful are small enough to tuck in your pocket—and
it is important to use them regularly and honestly to calculate how
many calories are taken in during the course of the day.

It is necessary to cut your intake of calories to 1,200 to 1,600
calories per day in order to achieve a weight loss of even one
pound a week. Although cutting down to this level theoretically
should result in greater and more rapid weight loss, at the start of
a diet the individual's metabolism usually becomes more efficient.
Although he feels that he is doing the same amount of activity as
he did before he commenced dieting, he actually burns fewer calories per day. This is a safety mechanism that appears to have been
designed to preserve the human race during times of famine, but
is inconvenient for those who now wish to lose weight.

For some individuals it may be as efficient to eliminate certain foods entirely from the diet and to limit others rather than to
calculate the intake of calories daily. The net effect of either
method is to cut calorie intake below that which is needed; in this
way the body will burn its stored fat and a slimmer individual will
emerge.

RATIONAL FOOD SELECTION

A good diet must be specific about what foods may not be
eaten; moreover, if the goal is to reduce the risk of heart disease,
the reducing diet must also avoid foods that are high in fat and
cholesterol. In order to do both—thus insuring a sensible reduction
in both weight and cholesterol levels—it is necessary to emphasize
foods that are low in calories and fat, but satisfying in effect. A
rational diet, then, depends heavily on fowl, fish, and lean red
meat; it directs the use of vegetables and fruit rather than starchy
prepared foods and allows a great deal of leeway in food selection.

In the main dish category, you will concentrate on the white
meat of fowl. Turkey, for example, is low in cholesterol and calories; it has the advantage of being a somewhat festive bird while
it is comparatively low in cost. Chicken is also low in calories and
saturated fat. And chicken fat, rendered from the skin and fat
which should never be eaten, is remarkably low in saturated fat
and contains far less cholesterol than most other animal fats. It can
be used occasionally to flavor certain vegetables and other foods.

(Chicken fat is also a good example of how to test for type of fat content: chicken fat and other unsaturated fats liquefy at room temperature, while butter and hydrogenated fats soften but do not turn to liquid.)

Duck is a more fatty fowl, somewhat higher in calories but relatively low in cholesterol. When fairly well cooked, with most of the fat drained out, duck can be included in the diet for variety. The kitchen of a famous diet spa revealed their secret of low-calorie duck. Before being served the fowl is carved and each portion placed on a piece of stale bread. Popped under the broiler for a few minutes, the bread absorbs whatever fat is left after roasting. Discard the bread and serve a good crisp piece of diet duck, garnished with orange slices or cherries for a good diet "company" meal.

It is not very sensible to reduce the size of your main dish serving too drastically, since it ordinarily provides your main source of protein. You will, of course, eat the same size serving that a nondieter would, even smaller if the portions in your house are larger than a quarter of a medium-sized chicken. It is a common mistake of dieters to increase the amount of permitted food far above what they would normally eat.

Any kind of fish is excellent on a diet. If you select a fatty fish like shad broil it, but other varieties can be baked or lightly sautéd in oil. Avoid deep frying or heavy crumb or batter coatings. In order to keep cholesterol and saturated fats to a minimum avoid the butter that is sometimes used quite unnecessarily to flavor fish. Try a squeeze of lemon juice instead, or a light coating of olive oil if a drier fish is to be broiled. Try baking your fish in a sauce made of tomato juice that has been seasoned and simmered with chopped onions, celery, and green pepper. (You can prepare this sauce ahead of time and keep it in your refrigerator for use on fish, chicken, or veal.) Fish is a good source of polyunsaturated oil and should be eaten whenever possible. Shellfish is relatively low in calories but significantly higher in a substance similar to cholesterol and should be eaten less frequently.

Canned fishes, such as salmon, tuna, or sardines, can be eaten freely, especially those that are packed in water rather than in oil. If you cannot enjoy the water-packed variety, be sure to drain the oil well. If you use water-packed fishes, try this tip supplied by the chef at an expensive spa. Drain well and season with lemon juice, pepper, chopped onion, or celery if desired. Then moisten with a dab of plain yogurt. Yogurt used in this way is a tangy, low-calorie, low-cholesterol substitute for mayonnaise.

Salmon and tuna can be eaten in salads or straight from the can, surrounded with greens and vegetables that you should be certain to eat. If they are used in casseroles, care should be taken to avoid adding too much in the way of high-calorie fillers—potatoes, rice, noodles, or cream soups.

Although fish and fowl should constitute the dieter's main sources of protein, there will be times when only a piece of good red meat will do. Try to limit these meals to no more than two or three times a week and be sure to remove all the fat you can see. If you choose a steak you are courting diet disaster if you consume the twelve or sixteen ounces that some restaurants consider a good-size serving. Eat your steak at home (it's far cheaper) and limit your portion to a moderate six or eight ounces. Cut off the fat prior to cooking, and broil well, one side at a time, to be sure that all the fat drips off. Whether it is rare or well done depends on your taste, although a certain amount of cooking is necessary to remove the fat that is marbled through the red meat. At today's prices it is probably wise to eat steak only once a week, and then only in a moderate-sized portion. The reason for this is that a twelve-ounce piece of well-marbled meat can easily run 1,000 calories or more, an astronomical price both financially and physically.

A meat that can be included a few times a week is veal, a lean meat which is similar in taste to white meat fowl. All visible fat should be removed and care should be taken not to prepare veal in sauces that are high in both calories and cholesterol. Ground veal patties are a good low-fat substitute for the ground beef hamburger. If you include lamb in your diet for variety, make it the spring or young grade since the older animal is high in saturated fat and cholesterol. Lamb should be broiled or oven roasted after all visible fat has been trimmed.

Pork products are very high in saturated fat so no bacon, ham, sausage, or pork should be eaten on a diet. Delicatessen meats such as hot dogs and smoked products such as bologna and salami should also be avoided. The fat content of hot dogs in this country is enormous—up to a third of the weight is currently permitted to be fat. Since a great deal of the rest is cereal filler, dieters can avoid hot dogs on several counts.

The common hamburger should also be approached warily on a rational diet. Unless you take the trouble to select a good lean piece of round steak and watch carefully while the butcher grinds it for you, it is likely to be high in fat. For real red meat enjoyment, you will be better off to enjoy your weekly steak. The hamburgers at the fast-food operations probably contain even more fat than you would buy in a pound of regular meat. If you find yourself at one of these counters try mopping the meat patty with the bread and then discarding the bun, another calorie reducer, or probably better yet, select the fish sandwich, discard the bread, and flake off the deep-fried crust.

Embellish your meat with vegetables in large amounts. Except for the starchy ones, all vegetables are excellent on a diet. Limit your intake of potatoes, corn, beans, and rice but feel free to include generous amounts of asparagus, broccoli, carrots, celery, cauliflower, cucumber, lettuce, mushrooms, parsley, summer squash, spinach, and tomatoes. Eat them raw in salads, or cooked without butter as a hot dish.

Salads in general should be featured; they give a lot of chewing satisfaction and aid in avoiding the constipation that sometimes plagues people when they begin to eat less food than they are accustomed to. An attractive salad packs a lot of satisfaction into a colorful package that is low in calories and cholesterol. You will be careful, though, with salad dressing. Consider yourself fortunate if you can enjoy a salad dressed only with lemon, or vinegar, or salt. If you must have a little bit of oil on your salad be certain that it is a clear oil high in polyunsaturates (safflower, soy, corn, or other vegetable oils) and try to limit its use to no more than a teaspoonful or two. Avoid mayonnaise and the commerically prepared creamy salad dressings, for they are high in both cholesterol and calories.

Be careful too with the large chef-type salads available in restaurants. Although they may be listed under specialties for dieters, they are often filled with ham, cheese, bacon bits, and other goodies that add calories. If you order a salad like this, be sure to pick and choose carefully. Eat the vegetables and fish, but avoid the crackers, the rich and creamy cheeses, and the delicatessen meats that add so much color—and so many calories. Cheese dressings should also be avoided, since they are usually high in both calories and cholesterol.

Other foods to be avoided are the rich cheeses and butter. Hard cheese may be enjoyed to the extent of about four ounces a week, but cream cheese and rich dessert cheeses are much too high in calories. Replace butter with corn oil margarine for polyunsaturates, and drink only skimmed or buttermilk. Low-fat cottage cheese is an excellent diet food, as is farmer cheese. Plain yogurt is useful on a diet. Mix it with farmer cheese for a creamy cheese that is reduced in calories, or try it slightly sweetened with sugar and honey as a low-fat topping for fruit or desserts. The fruited yogurts are high in sugar and calories so remember to concentrate on imaginative uses for the plain variety.

Some successful dieters find it helpful to take coffee and tea with sugar. Although higher in calories than nonnutritive sweeteners, for many people the teaspoonful of sugar is more satisfying and provides the lift they need, especially between meals, to continue dieting. Again moderation is the rule: no more than a teaspoonful or two of sugar per cup of hot beverage, with total sugar intake in beverages limited to no more than ten teaspoonfuls per day. As many cups of hot tea or coffee as desired can be taken within the limit of ten teaspoons of sugar per day. Use no cream in your coffee, substituting skim milk or small amounts of powdered lightener. This use of hot beverages with sugar can be a satisfying aid to long-term dieting.

Your summertime beverages will revolve around the new calorie-free diet sodas, a really remarkable advance in diet foods. Be careful, though, to avoid the sugar-added varieties that contain up to 8 calories per *ounce,* a whopping 64 calories per eight-ounce glass! These drinks should not be called diet sodas at all and have no place in your daily regimen. You can enjoy a cool and refreshing diet dessert drink by mixing the low-calorie diet sodas with nonfat dry milk solids, some ice cubes, and some fresh fruit. Whirl it up in the blender for a thick milkshake-type drink that is excellent for dieters and nondieters alike.

Alcohol should be limited or avoided altogether, since it contains a great many calories and little nutrition. If a drink is absolutely necessary, have it with ice, water, or plain club soda, and do not even consider having the pretzels or nuts that accompany the drink. Beer is absolutely prohibited on any diet, and all alcohol intake should be limited to no more than two shots in a twenty-four-hour period.

Baked goods and other starches must be approached carefully. If you are one of those people who are disoriented without at least one slice of bread a day, try having it toasted with cottage cheese for a good breakfast. Choose a bread that is enriched, toast it to increase its chewability, and enjoy it in limited quantities of no more than two or three slices a day depending on your needs.

The wife of one of my successful dieters invested some time ago in a gadget that allows her to slice bread and rolls lengthwise, creating two thin slices from one piece of bread. She uses it to thinly slice bagels into fourths, and reports that her husband has enjoyed a half of a toasted bagel for years in the belief that he was eating the whole thing.

You will not even purchase pretzels, potato chips, or snack crackers of any kind. They are high in starch and fillers and calories and extremely low in everything else. "Small" foods packing a lot of calories into a little corpus should be avoided since you could easily consume half of your day's allowance in one evening in front of the television set.

Avoid pastry and cookies of all kinds. There is no such thing as a diet cookie; even when it is labeled as such it is high in carbohydrate, fat, and calories. Dietetic baked goods may be fine for diabetics who are concerned mainly with their sugar intake, but for the ordinary weight-loss diet they are still too high in calories.

Your desserts will revolve around fruits. If you cannot get fresh fruit, try the new canned varieties packed in water or their own juice. They are usually excellent and the caloric value is significantly less than for those packed in heavy syrup. Some fruits have more calories than others (bananas, cherries, apples), but all are useful because they are satisfying. They are the answer to the dessert question because they are attractive and can be chewed with a great deal of sensual pleasure. Consult your calorie counter for relative contents, but in general if you concentrate on crunchy fruits and citrus fruits you will keep your intake in control. Good apples crunch, pears crunch, and if you listen closely even plums and cantaloupe crunch. Mushy fruits like bananas, figs, and grapes do not crunch and are higher in calories; approach grapes warily for a bunch of grapes can easily provide most of your meal's calories. Grapefruit, although it works no miracles that I can see, is good on a diet because it takes a lot of time to eat and provides a lot of Vitamin C for its caloric content. Enjoy it with sugar or salt or pop it under the broiler with a glaze of honey on top. Either way it is an excellent first course or dessert.

Dried or preserved fruits are much higher in calories than fresh fruit and should be avoided. They are usually full of sugar and may entice the dieter to eat far in excess of his needs—try eating one raisin, for instance.

Eggs, although high in cholesterol, are a good source of protein and a valuable aid to some dieters. If you have no known lipid abnormalities, and if your family history is relatively free of evidence of premature heart disease, then you may have one egg three times a week. If you have honestly cut down on your intake of baked goods, you have probably reduced your egg intake markedly. Adding several eggs for breakfast or for some variety at lunch should not increase your cholesterol intake beyond that which can be handled by normal adults. Prepare your egg without fat, in the top of a double boiler for exceptional scrambled eggs or in a coated pan that allows you to slide a lightly fried egg out without a lot of grease.

The coffee break can be a perilous time for dieters, especially if their co-workers have enriched the occasion with pastries or breakfast rolls. Be firm about refusing, or you will find that you have added another meal to your day's pattern. If you use some sugar in your hot beverage instead of saccharine, the break will be more satisfying and you will be better able to make it through the morning to lunchtime.

Late in the afternoon most dieters find that they need a pickup of some kind. Coffee or tea with sugar or bouillon should get you going again, with a small piece of fruit or hard cheese added if you are really dragging. If you are going to have a drink, enjoy it before dinner. It is relaxing and helps to cut your appetite for sweets somewhat.

Early in the course of your diet it is valuable to spend a few minutes at the end of the day recording the foods you have eaten; by using one of the many calorie counters available you can easily determine the total number of calories for that day. If the count exceeds 1,800, it may be necessary to be less liberal with your intake of starchy vegetables or high-calorie fruits.

In general, begin by consciously substituting lower calorie, more nutritious foods for the more fattening ones: clear soup for cream soup, green salad or cole slaw for potato salad or baked beans, fruit for pastry, low-calorie beverages for high; fish or chicken for red meat. These choices will soon become habitual and you will be on your way to a lifelong program of weight control.

DIETING IN RESTAURANTS

I have little patience with people who claim that they cannot diet because they must eat out a great deal, and I am positively hostile to those who dine in restaurants loudly bemoaning the fact that they are on a diet. The fact is that for some people restaurant meals are easier to limit because they are denied access to the kitchen and must be content with whatever is served.

Furthermore, if you think for a moment about when you eat most in the course of a restaurant meal, you will realize that it is the extras that are sneaky, not the meal itself. My own observation is that you eat most of the fattening food *after* the waiter has taken your order, but *before* he arrives with the meal itself.

The rational dieter will thus enter a good restaurant determined to enjoy the meal itself. He will ignore the roll basket; if there is a relish tray on the table he will enjoy the raw vegetables but go very easy on the olives because they are in the "little" fruit category and pack a lot of calories into a small corpus. An assertive dieter will persuade the waiter to serve his salad almost at once and he will busy himself with that while everyone else is going through the hot breads. He will drink as little as possible, especially at lunch when his lowered food intake will increase the soporific or sleep-inducing effects of the alcohol.

At either lunch or dinner the dieter would do well to avoid restaurant soups. Most are quite starchy—that thick smooth effect is usually the result of cornstarch—and even clear soups can be high in fat. Select an appetizer that is low in calories and substantial enough so that you can ignore the crackers served with it. Cold seafood cocktails are nice if you can forego the oyster crackers. Chopped liver, if it is served without fat, should be eaten without crackers or rye bread, unless you are cheating. Order your vegetables without butter, quietly please because nothing is more boring than someone else's diet.

If the main dish portion is much larger than you are accustomed to, by all means cut it in half and take the rest home for another meal. Do not be shy about doggie bags—at today's prices they are the ultimate in chic—and do not feel that you must finish everything on your plate. If you are finished, signal the busboy to remove your plate by quietly placing your knife and fork upside down at the top of the plate. Most adults are conditioned to finish everything on their plate and the best antidote for this is to have it removed.

Dessert should simply not be ordered in a restaurant unless you are having your cheating meal. If they can supply a piece of melon or grapefruit, fine, but anything more than that is superfluous. You have probably eaten more than your fill and a good cup of coffee or tea should get you through any restaurant meal without going off your diet.

CHEATING IN RESTAURANTS

Most successful dieters choose to have their cheating meals in restaurants, in this way enjoying an evening out while they are fulfilling all of their food fantasies. In fact, the secret of effective cheating is to have the things about which you have fantasized during a week of fairly honest dieting.

If you have been having dreams about steak and mashed potatoes this is the time to enjoy them. Trim the fat from the meat and go easy on the bread and butter if they have not played a part in your dreams. If it is dessert that you yearn for, select a fairly sensible main dish but go wild at the end of the meal. The secret, of course, is to cheat only with the things you really want and then on a really large scale. In this way you will accomplish something useful with your cheating meal; you will avoid the guilt of having gorged on stuff you really did not want and you will be able to go back to your diet without regrets.

VITAMINS

Every diet requires some restriction on food intake and may result in mild vitamin or mineral deficiencies. Even though a rational diet supplies most of the vegetables, fruit, and protein sources you need for good nutrition, it is possible that the foods you select may lack some important vitamins. I suggest, therefore, that everyone who goes on a diet for any length of time supplement it with a vitamin preparation.

Try to select a vitamin tablet that is well balanced, providing the minimum daily requirement of everything you need. And do not skimp on the price you pay for vitamins. Although all labels are required to list exactly what the preparation contains, vitamins can vary widely in other respects. For example, if the pills are not formulated properly the vitamins they contain may deteriorate long before you will have used up the tablets. This is false economy; spend the money you save on ice cream and other snacks forbidden on your diet to buy the vitamin product of a good drug house. If you take a good multivitamin once a day, nutritional deficiency will be last on the list of things you need to worry about.

SOME AIDS TO DIETING

When you are on a diet, it is important that you increase the amount of sleep you get. Dieting does not combine well with fatigue, and when you are tired you simply lack the will power to keep from eating. When you are very tired you may seek the energy you need in a bit of extra food; if you have work to do you may find that eating a great deal gives you the jolt you need to get something accomplished. Whether this is true or only an impression shared by a lot of people, the fact is that fatigue is both trying and fattening.

Go to bed at a decent hour—thereby shortening your evening snacking time, another plus on any diet—and try to get at least seven or eight hours of sleep a night. This is especially important for active people who sometimes find that they gain weight even though they work hard. If you increase the amount of rest you get while you decrease your food intake you will find dieting a much easier task.

Seek to be as emotionally stable as possible. Equilibrium is a great aid in dieting. If you are under a great deal of stress, wait for a time when things have settled down and then start your diet. When you are changing your status—marrying or divorcing, changing jobs, moving, or undertaking new responsibilities—do not begin to diet. Eat moderately if you can, but wait until a more propitious time to start your serious dieting.

It is also unwise to embark on a reducing diet when you are ill. If you have so much as a cold do not start a diet. If you are on a diet and become sick with a fever or other systemic illness that reveals itself with objective signs, let up on the diet for a few days. This is also a form of stress, and it does not pay to diet when the body is fighting off infection or some other physical insult. Dieting itself is a form of stress, and you should be in as good physical shape as is possible before you undertake this additional strain.

KEEPING THE WEIGHT OFF

The diet described here is a rational meal plan that represents a decrease in caloric intake for most people. If it is followed carefully, most moderately active adults will lose one to two pounds each week. And this will be a stable loss, one that you can count on week after week as long as you stay on the diet.

When you have attained the look you like and the scale confirms that you have indeed lost the weight you desired, this is not the time to stop dieting. Remember, rational people who tend to gain weight know that they must maintain some form of dietary control if they are to remain comfortable and slim. Gaining back weight lost after a considerable struggle is irrational in the extreme.

So you will not celebrate your new figure by immediately eating everything you wish. Relax a little bit on portion control, eating an entire steak, for example, if this gives you great pleasure. Add one or two slices of bread to your daily intake, or alternate with a potato at the evening meal. You should continue to avoid pastries since once this habit is broken it is best left unmourned; if desserts are your downfall, add a scoop of ice cream to your cantaloupe, or enjoy a cone with the kids in the summer.

Continue to be careful at coffee breaks or you will soon find that you have added an unnecessary meal composed of many empty calories. You should always be wary of butter, cream, and rich cheeese since these are a source of cholesterol as well as of calories. Use the margarine that proudly lists liquid oil first on its label and add only a small amount of whole milk to your coffee if you really cannot abide the skimmed variety. Adult males and postmenopausal women should never have more than three eggs a week, even when not trying to lose weight.

By observing these few simple rules you can remain on a low-calorie, low-cholesterol diet that is fairly easy to live with. Remember, though, if you want to maintain your new lowered body weight you can add only about 600 calories each day. If you want to know exactly how little this is, consult your calorie counter since a piece of pie, one dessert, and a whole steak can easily amount to more than 600 calories *each*.

You have worked too hard to unwittingly find yourself on the dangerous seesaw of repeated weight loss and subsequent gain. Keep an eye on the scale at your weekly weigh in. For the first two weeks or so after the strict dieting ends you may still show a loss of one or two pounds. Do not be too elated by this for by the third week the drop will be much less and by the fourth week your weight will have stabilized.

This is now a dangerous time, for if you do not cut back at once by week seven or eight you may find that you have gained a pound or so. When the weekly weigh-in shows a gain of two pounds or more, serious measures must be taken to stop the trend at once. Cut back to your dieting regimen, eliminating the extras that helped add the weight. And watch the scale carefully until it shows that you have returned once more to the weight that you consider ideal.

In this way, by being ever watchful, you can use these successive approximations to maintain a good weight on a fairly comfortable pattern of eating. After the triumph of a successful diet you do not want to sacrifice your hard-won slenderness to a few high-calorie foods, eaten for the most part unconsciously and unknowingly.

In summary, then, to diet successfully:

1. Choose a realistic goal.
2. Personalize your diet with foods you prefer and a meal schedule that suits you.
3. Count the calories you consume each day, using one of the many calorie counters available.
4. For vigorous dieting, eat 1,200 to 1,400 calories per day; for moderate dieting, 1,600 calories per day.

5. Eliminate the empty calories of snacks and "junk" foods; be careful with coffee breaks.
6. Expect to be hungry, but just because you are hungry do not assume that you are dieting effectively. Count calories honestly—not wishfully.
7. Do not cut out sugar in coffee and tea. The pickup is useful and effective at the small cost of 17 calories per level teaspoon.
8. Do not have fattening foods in the house.
9. Weigh yourself once a week.
10. Do not expect to lose much in the first two weeks and do not get discouraged. A good weight loss is one to two pounds each week.
11. Select foods that are low in saturated fats.
12. Do *not* increase the portion size of acceptable foods just because they are high in protein and low in fat and carbohydrate; rather, *cut* the portion size of everything you eat.
13. Learn to cheat correctly: admit that you are cheating and do it only once each week—then cheat big!
14. Get plenty of sleep; do not attempt to diet when under physical or emotional stress.
15. Once you have achieved your goal, dieting is *not* over. Maintain sound eating habits and be ever watchful for a weight gain of more than one or two pounds.

Chapter 10

Exercise: Its Role in Good Heart Health

The arguments in favor of exercise as a means of reducing one's risk of heart attack are very tempting. What could be more pleasant than to forget dark words about hypertension or the high fat content of the typical American diet and just take to the tennis courts, the ski slopes, or even the gym in the name of good cardiovascular health? Enthusiasts of every persuasion—physicians, superannuated gymnasts, all-round athletes, and devotees of one exercise form or another—all get into print easily with articles, books, devices, and programs that promise long life and freedom from heart attacks to those who jog, drill, run in place, or just work hard.

The truth is that exercise can be of considerable benefit in an all-encompassing cardiac conditioning program; like every other prescription in medicine, however, exercise must be used sensibly and according to directions that take into account the individual's medical history as well as the climate, both social and meteorological, in which he exercises.

Moreover, like so many other elements in the equation of good heart health, the role of exercise as a coronary risk factor is not completely understood. That is, there is no scientifically acceptable way of "proving" that increasing any individual's exercise level decreases that individual's risk of heart attack. There are, however, some important studies that strongly suggest that *regular* exertion may indeed confer some kind of protection against heart disease. And there are other studies—anecdotal and controlled—reporting that regular exercise does indeed confer an increased sense of well-being that must be equated with good mental and physical health. In addition, of course, exercise is the only one of the coronary risk factors whose modification can be cited as pleasurable and positive, allowing the individual to develop new interests and new methods for using leisure time while at the same time helping to condition his heart and cardiovascular system.

Interestingly enough, people who positively recoil at the idea of changing their dietary habits or who go into a blue funk at the thought of giving up cigarettes can usually be counted upon to jump feet first into the most recently publicized form of physical conditioning. Unfortunately, this is exactly the *wrong* way to even think about exercise as a coronary risk factor, and for this reason I will present some fairly firm cautionary advice in this chapter. Rational adults who wish to increase their level of activity with a view toward looking and feeling better are well advised to regard exercise as a prescription just like any other. Directions concerning the use of exercise should be carefully followed and any untoward effects should be noted and reported to the physician.

Exercise is also a prescription whose application must be determined by several extraneous factors. Certainly the basic state of the individual's health must be determined—by the physician who best knows his background—before any conditioning program is begun. Furthermore, the patient must temper even these directions with his own good judgment concerning the atmosphere, both internal and external, in which he exercises: what is perfectly safe when the temperature is 70 degrees may be lethal at 92 degrees or on a cold and windy February day. It is only sensible to forego any strenuous activity when you have a cold or are otherwise not up to par.

These matters are discussed in detail in the following pages (exercise conditioning for the postcoronary patient is covered in Volume II), but first I shall present the evidence on behalf of increased exercise as a factor in reducing your risk of heart attack.

THE CASE FOR EXERCISE

The classic study suggesting that increased activity may indeed confer some kind of cardiac protection was done in England in the 1950s. J. N. Morris and his co-workers, investigating the health records of employees of the London Transport System, were struck by the difference in coronary disease rates between the men who worked as conductors and those who worked as drivers. The conductors were required to move about constantly, running up and down the stairs of the double-deck vehicles collecting fares and looking after the passengers, while the drivers spent almost all of their working day sitting in place, their only real exertion being to turn the wheel of the bus and argue with other drivers.

The researchers were struck by their finding that the incidence of heart attacks among conductors was only half that found among drivers. This led to a study that compared postal employees who walked their route with those who worked as clerks; again there was an increase in mortality from coronary heart disease in those with the more sedentary occupations, suggesting that the considerable amount of walking done by the postmen may have conferred some protection against heart attacks.

In this country, W. J. Zukel studied a group of men living in the rural areas of North Dakota, seeking to compare heart disease rates among farmers with nonfarmers who shared the same living conditions. This research noted specifically that men who engaged in heavy work one to two hours daily had an incidence of coronary disease that was only 18 per cent of those who did no heavy work, a striking finding.

A study of railroad men disclosed that those who worked outdoors as switchmen had a significantly lower rate of mortality from arteriosclerotic heart disease than that of men who worked inside as railroad clerks or ticket sellers. In Evans County, Georgia, sharecroppers who actually worked the farms were found to have an incidence of coronary heart disease only one-third that of the farm owners. Small farm owners who presumably did a great deal of the heavy work themselves, again, had an incidence of coronary disease only one-third of those who owned large farms, and men who reported doing heavy work full time had only 17 percent the heart disease rate of those who did no heavy work at all.

This kind of study was repeated in Israel, where men who lived on collective farms and did considerable physical work were found to have a heart attack rate only one third of those who lived under the same conditions but had more sedentary jobs.

S. Shapiro and his co-workers studied a group of men aged thirty-five to sixty-four who participated in the Health Insurance Plan of New York. They found only half the incidence of myocardial infarctions among those who were either very active or intermediately active when compared with the group reporting the least amount of physical activity. Mortality from coronary heart disease was also strikingly different; only 20 to 25 percent of the men in the active groups died when suffering heart attacks as compared to the least active group.

One of the few prospective studies was reported in 1973 by J. N. Morris and his colleagues. They followed a large group of 17,000 male executive-grade civil servants, aged forty to sixty-four, over a five-year period starting in 1968. Participants were asked to complete a questionnaire detailing their activities for a specific working day, a Friday, and for the Saturday following when they presumably followed their usual schedule of leisure activity. Over the follow-up period 232 men suffered a clinical attack of coronary disease, and each of these was matched with two other subjects who had remained essentially healthy. Among the men with coronary disease there was a significantly lowered rate of strenuous activity during the sample leisure period when compared with the more active men of the healthy control group.

AND WHAT DOES IT ALL MEAN?

These data provide some fascinating information, and some equally fascinating questions. All of these studies suggest that heavy physical activity, taken regularly as part of one's daily work or leisure, may confer on the individual some degree of protection from coronary heart disease. But it must also be noted that people who engage in heavy physical activity most often do so from choice and hence might be constitutionally stronger, or otherwise "different," to start with. Moreover, occupations not involved with a high level of physical activity are frequently associated with considerable emotional stress that may also interact with other coronary risk factors such as cigarette smoking, obesity, and hypertension.

But the evidence in favor of increasing one's exercise level in order to reduce the risk of heart attack may actually be supported by this latter association. Well-documented studies have shown that increased levels of physical activity are of demonstrable benefit in the control of the other coronary risk factors. Increased exercise, judiciously used, helps to lower blood pressure and also appears to interact in the control of lipid levels of the blood; studies done before and after increased exercise showed a marked lowering of triglycerides, one of the blood fat constituents thought to increase the risk of heart attack. Since it is difficult—and very foolish—to continue to smoke while on an exercising program, this risk factor is also favorably influenced, as is obesity, exercise always having been considered an effective adjunct to weight control.

Stress as a coronary risk factor is more difficult to pin down and measure, but there is no question that proper exercise can aid in discharging the accumulated tensions that appear to characterize the Type-A or coronary-prone personality. A recent study suggests that exercise is a far more potent antianxiety measure than meprobamate, one of the most widely used tranquilizer drugs. Psychological tests following exercise show a marked decrease in anxiety; the well-known relaxation reported by golfers and tennis players is probably related to this discharge of anxiety and tension.

Thus, although no one to date can "prove" that increasing exercise levels directly decreases the risk of heart attack, there is ample evidence to conclude that regular exercise is a pleasant and worthwhile part of any cardiovascular fitness program.

THE PHYSIOLOGY OF EXERCISE

Although the beneficial effects of exercise have been noted, the exact mechanism of its action is not yet completely understood. One interpretation of the role of exercise in cardiac protection holds that physical activity demands an increase in the work of the heart. This may enlarge the coronary arteries to such an extent that, when atherosclerosis does develop, it takes significantly more of the disease to close the artery. Although this is a reasonable hypothesis, it has not yet been proved in humans.

Another theory holds that exercise may stimulate the development of collateral circulation, the additional vessels that parallel the main lines of supply to the heart. When blood supply to the heart is cut off by a heart attack or coronary occlusion, these collateral vessels may be able to provide enough nourishment to avoid the damage that would be caused by total occlusion. No proof of this has been demonstrated, but the collateral circulation argument was invoked most strongly to explain former President Eisenhower's almost complete recovery from his heart attacks. His lifelong pattern of regular exercise appeared to have conditioned his heart to the point where it withstood several serious infarctions. A recent study supported this concept. Heart attacks were created in two groups of rats that were similar except that one group had been exercized by swimming every day for about a month. The exercised rats had significantly less heart damage than the others. The experimenters considered this result to be attributable to an increase in vascularity in the hearts of the exercised animals.

Another school holds that regular exercise strengthens the heart in the same way that it would any other muscle. During vigorous exercise the heart is required to participate by increasing the blood flow to the body, conditioning the heart muscle in the same way that leg exercises condition the leg muscles. An area of damage in a physiologically robust heart would probably be tolerated better than in an organ that is less well conditioned.

All of these hypotheses are interesting and reasonable but none has yet been proved in an intact human. The studies that are documented, however, provide striking proof that exercise can be effective in lowering the blood pressure and reducing the triglyceride levels of the blood. Other research has demonstrated that physical activity reduces the tendency of the blood to clot, a promising avenue for continued research since blood clots play an important role in the development of strokes and heart attacks. In addition, regular exercise has been shown to increase the level of high density lipoprotein in the blood. Higher blood levels of this lipoprotein have been correlated with a lessened tendency toward development of coronary disease. This lipoprotein may act as a scavenger removing cholesterol from the coronary vessel wall before atherosclerotic plaques have developed into occlusive lesions.

The other demonstrable results of exercise have to do with its positive effects on the response of the heart rate to stress of any kind and on its level of activity at rest. Individuals who are well conditioned have a lowered resting heart rate, evidence of increased efficiency of the heart and further evidence that the heart is pumping more blood with each stroke. This lowered resting heart rate is one of the main benefits of cardiac conditioning.

The work of the heart and its oxygen requirement at rest are also reduced. A conditioned and efficient heart can increase the volume it pumps with just a moderate rise in rate. Well-conditioned people appear to respond to stress in a well-modulated way. The heart rate rises relatively slowly and the sympathetic nervous system is less stimulated by any degree of emotional or physical exertion. Exercise also appears to provide a greater amount of reserve capacity that can be called upon under severe conditions.

For all of these reasons, proved and hypothesized, it may be that people who are well conditioned by regular physical activity can avoid the more serious consequences of atherosclerosis and delay the onset of some forms of coronary heart disease. Exercise is a pleasant and rewarding activity, and its beneficial effect on the risk of developing heart disease has to be seen as a dividend.

DYNAMIC VERSUS ISOMETRIC EXERCISE

Before I go into the details of a conditioning program, please note that only dynamic exercise—the kind that involves movement —is of benefit to the cardiovascular system. These exercises require that the heart beat faster to increase cardiac output and stimulating a vigorous increase in heart rate is the desired end of any conditioning program. Blood flow throughout the body is stepped up by dynamic exercise, and there is usually only a moderate increase in blood pressure.

Isometric exercise, on the other hand, is concerned mostly with building muscles—in contrast to the qualities of building stamina and endurance in dynamic exercise. Weight lifting, push-ups, chin-ups, and pushing and pulling of any kind are all forms of isometric exercise, and none is considered helpful in conditioning the heart or cardiovascular system. Moreover, isometric exercise works by tightening or contracting the muscles, an effort which significantly raises the blood pressure. Sometimes the rise in blood pressure is sudden and the inordinate stress placed on the heart may have dire results. An isometric contraction of any muscle may actually decrease blood flow as a result of the constricting effect on the blood vessels. For cardiac conditioning, isometric exercise should be avoided and dynamic activities emphasized.

There are many daily activities that are primarily isometric and precipitate angina or other symptoms of cardiac insufficiency in people with overt or unknown coronary disease. For example, snow shoveling, a push-pull-lift form of isometric exercise, frequently precedes a sudden heart attack in men who have subclinical coronary disease. People with known coronary disease are also warned not to carry heavy loads or to keep their arms overhead for any length of time—two essentially isometric activities.

HOW TO CONDITION THE HEART

For the serious symptom-free adult with several hours to spare each week, a structured exercise program may be the most effective method of conditioning the heart. (A program of moderate exercise for cardiac rehabilitation following a heart attack is given in Volume II.)

The first step in this or any other exercise program is to obtain your physician's approval. This is especially important if you have ever had an abnormal electrocardiogram, or if you have ever had any symptoms of chest pain, shortness of breath, joint pain, diabetes, or high blood pressure. If you are more than twenty pounds overweight or smoke more than one pack of cigarettes each day, it is probably a good idea to see your physician before embarking on any program of vigorous activity.

The reason for this caution is that an effective conditioning program works by raising the heart rate to about 75 percent of the maximum of which it is capable. Since this is two to two and one-half times the resting rate, conditioning does require considerable exertion. (The rule of thumb is that the maximum heart rate expected in an individual is approximately 220 beats per minute minus the individual's age: a fifty-year old man is expected to have a maximal heart rate of about 170 and a twenty-five-year old a maximal heart rate of about 195. In an exercise conditioning program featuring 75 percent of maximum, these individuals would work up to heart rates of about 135 and 148 beats per minute, respectively.) Moreover, it is necessary to maintain this increased rate for ten to fifteen minutes several times each week in order to achieve any kind of cardiac conditioning effect. This is hard work; for this reason, it is necessary to know that you are in fairly good shape before commencing an exercise program.

Your physician may want to take both a resting and an exercise ECG. He will also probably take a history of your health status and perhaps draw some blood for laboratory determination of any underlying conditions.

EXERCISE CONDITIONING

With your physician's approval, and assured of your own good judgment in determining goals, you can embark on an exercise conditioning program in one of several ways. I would like to recommend that you ask your local heart association about supervised exercise programs that may be available in your area. Cardiac conditioning programs are sometimes sponsored by medical centers or may be offered by the local YMCA or other community center. While I cannot comment on each program, my observation in general is that they are usually well run and well constructed for maximum effectiveness. By enrolling in an established program, you can take advantage of the group's expertise in what may be a new field to you. Moreover, working out in a group is easier for many people than exercising alone. The support of others may also supply the motivation you need to continue your program long after it has ceased to be novelty. Supervised programs for men and women who have had heart attacks usually feature the constant electrocardiographic monitoring of the heart, although any institutional conditioning program should be prepared to cope with any untoward effects.

HOW TO TAKE YOUR PULSE

Each session of your exercise conditioning program should consist of a ten- to fifteen-minute period of activity that achieves the heart rate that you have designated as your goal. Except in rare instances, pulse rate is the same as heart rate so it is a fairly simple matter to determine heart rate by taking your pulse. The pulse rate can be taken easily at any of several points on the upper body. Try placing two or three fingers firmly against the temple or on the thumb side of the thick tendons on the inside surface of the wrist. Since it is necessary to partially close off the artery to feel the blood pulse through, you will have to press fairly firmly. Holding a watch with a sweep-second hand in the other hand, count the pulse for fifteen seconds. Multiply by four for a one-minute pulse determination. Most middle-aged adults will count a rate of 65 to 85 beats per minute at rest.

In either a supervised or self-administered program, the ideal conditioning is achieved by working out on three or four nonconsecutive days each week in fifteen- to twenty-minute sessions that are preceded and followed by short warm-up and cool-down periods. Since the pulse rate is a sensitive barometer of exertion that falls off almost immediately when activity stops, it is a good idea to take your pulse as soon as you have stopped exercising. You may also take it before you start.

Warm up for several minutes and then take your pulse. It will probably be less than three-quarters of the rate you are aiming for but it will give some idea of how vigorously you should work out in the next five minutes or so of your session. Proceed by working out vigorously for the next five to seven minutes and then taking your pulse as soon as you cease the activity. If it exceeds your target goal of 75 percent of maximum, then slow down; if it is less than your goal, continue the exercise more vigorously for a period *if you are not too tired.*

You must heed your built-in warning system to determine how early in your program you will attain the desired 75 percent of maximum heart rate. Conditioning means building up to desired goals and then working to maintain them. You can use your pulse rate determination to gauge how soon or how fast you will reach the target, but you must also heed your own feelings to stay out of trouble. As conditioning proceeds you will find that gradually more work is required to achieve the desired rate. This is evidence that your heart is being conditioned.

Incorporating exercise into one's daily activity requires only a good measure of common sense. For healthy adults with no symptoms of heart disease and for those whose physicians have given approval, the keynotes must be moderation and regularity. Far too often, middle-aged men who really should know better jump on the bandwagon of jogging or other strenuous exercise—with dire or unpleasant results. Or an enthusiastic exerciser may work out strenuously, once, and while massaging his aching muscles the next day wonder why he does not feel better. Only moderate exercise, regularly done, can achieve sound and effective conditioning.

It is heartening, however, that most people have a good built-in warning system, and when they rely on their own common sense it usually works very well. Exercise, like sex, should be enjoyed by everyone to his or her maximum level—no more and no less.

Because you enjoy your maximum level of activity, you will

be able to continue it over a long period of time, an essential factor in any kind of conditioning program. The goal of any exercise regimen is to develop new habits so that the pattern is continued long after the good intentions are forgotten and the resolutions like those made on New Year's Eve have vanished. It is thus essential that the activity be pleasant and fun to do with regularity over a long period of time.

CYCLE CONDITIONING

For those people who function better with a specific program, there are two easily available methods for exercise conditioning at home. In both methods the amount of exertion is determined by the individual's heart rate response as determined by taking the pulse. The goal is 75 percent of the age-predicted maximum for normal adults, about 150 beats per minute for a twenty-five-year-old man and about 130 for a fifty-year-old. When this level of exertion has been reached, it should be maintained for approximately fifteen minutes to achieve maximum conditioning effect.

One of the simplest home exercise programs involves the use of a stationary bicycle. The bicycle should be equipped with a speedometer or RPM meter and a method to increase the resistance. Try putting the bike in a room with a television set. In this way you can develop an easily followed routine, pedaling while you watch the evening news, for example. Television viewing makes the time go more pleasantly and also helps you to gauge the time you have spent at your program.

Set the resistance knob at a moderate level. After a two- to three-minute warm-up at a moderate two to three miles per hour, pedal for a few minutes at five to six miles per hour. Stop and immediately take your pulse. If it is lower than your individual target rate, increase the resistance to a higher setting and repeat the procedure. If your pulse rate measures higher than you desire, slow the pedaling speed to three to four miles an hour and take your pulse again. Once the speed and resistance level needed to achieve the desired pulse rate have been reached, continue to pedal until you have worked at the target rate for ten to fifteen minutes in all.

You will have to determine this at every second exercise session, setting the resistance knob and rates of speed at different levels because, as conditioning progresses successfully, you will have to increase the level of resistance and the rate of pedaling to attain the desired heart rate. This will also provide a measure of your progress in conditioning: when you are able to do more work at a lower heart rate you are achieving your conditioning goals.

WALKING PROGRAM

The same kind of conditioning program can be developed if it is convenient for you to walk long distances every day. As with bicycling, the goal is 75 percent of maximum age-predicted heart rate. The amount of heart rate elevation that you will experience is determined by the speed at which you walk. In people who are poorly conditioned, or out of shape at the start of their program, walking at a rate of three miles per hour (a mile and a half in thirty minutes) is usually sufficient to raise the heart rate to the desired level. A mile is approximately ten city blocks, but you can use your car's speedometer to determine the exact length of the course you wish to follow. Start by walking briskly and after about five minutes continue walking while you take your pulse. If the rate is higher than the desired level, slow down; if it measures lower than you wish, speed up your walking rate. Among younger people or those who are in good physical shape, walking even fairly briskly may not provide sufficient exertion to allow you to attain the target heart rate, and in this case jogging may be added to your program.

JOGGING

First I must warn that starting a program with jogging, especially if you are not in top condition, is dangerous. Jogging requires a great deal of exertion and the heart may rapidly reach a rate that is far higher than you desire. Only by working up to your goal slowly, and by adhering to the guideline of achieving 75 percent of maximum for ten to fifteen minutes and not beyond, can you add jogging to an exercise program with safety.

Jogging should never be added to an exercise program until after you have determined that very vigorous walking does not succeed in attaining the target heart rate. It is also a good idea to warm up first at each exercise session by walking briskly for several minutes; once you have begun to jog it is important to check your pulse rate five minutes or so after you start in order to be certain that it has not gone beyond the rate you are aiming for. You should do this every time you go out to jog because environmental conditions have a marked effect on cardiovascular responses. If it is very cold, very warm, or even very humid, the heart rate response will be higher for the same amount of work. If you are not well rested or are otherwise not feeling up to par, the heart rate will also go higher than you would expect.

The rule in any conditioning program is that you should not push yourself if you are not feeling well, if your response causes you any worry, or if there is even a question as to how you feel. No exercise program is completely safe, and if there is any question you should proceed cautiously and with the detailed advice of your physician.

At the end of any conditioning session, it is important to cool down, allowing a few minutes of slower activity to permit the blood circulation distribution to return gradually to resting levels. During exercise, more blood goes to the activated muscles. At rest and during normal activity, the blood flow is distributed differently and the shift must be allowed to occur gradually.

As conditioning progresses with moderation and regularity, you will feel an increased ability to achieve more. The amount of exertion required to achieve the target heart rate will gradually increase, but the rules concerning guidelines and taking the pulse should be followed continually to achieve maximum conditioning with safety.

EXERCISE AS PART OF DAILY LIVING

Human nature being what it is, I find it likely that only the best intentioned individuals will be able to continue this compulsive type of activity for an extended period of time. For myself and for most people, I believe that it is easier to develop patterns of subtly increased activity that are pleasant enough to maintain for many years and which do not require the expenditure of a great deal of time in essentially useless activity.

The easiest way to begin an informal exercise program is to adhere religiously to the principle of never riding when it is possible to walk. If you work in a high-rise building the corollary is never to take an elevator to go up one or down two flights of stairs. If you determine that you will achieve conditioning by increasing the amount of walking that you do each day, you can begin by getting into the habit of not using your car when you are going only five or six blocks from your home or office. If you commute by bus or train, you can increase your daily exercise by allowing enough time to get off a stop or two away from your office. By walking this added distance each day, you will add significantly to the amount of exercise you are able to achieve over a long period of time. As conditioning proceeds and you can do more with less effort, try getting off two or three stops away from your destination.

Once you have reached your office, you can forgo the elevator in favor of walking the stairs. Again you can increase the number of flights walked as conditioning proceeds, and you can also increase the speed with which you take the stairs. Try walking the stairs two at a time when you have achieved the goal of twenty or twenty-two steps in fifty seconds or less.

If you drive to work try leaving your car at a parking lot some distance from the office. That way you will add exercise both in the morning and evening. Take every opportunity that you can for increased walking; it is a healthful and inexpensive way to obtain the daily conditioning that you need. During your leisure time, try walking just for pleasure. In your neighborhood this might be a good way to get to know your neighbors or to walk the dog; in the city it is a pleasant means of getting from place to place without your car and of checking on the latest displays in the store windows. If you have children, walking might provide a good way of spending leisure time with them. On the weekends try a trip to the zoo or to some local attraction that allows you to walk while you observe the sights.

Although walking is easy and costs nothing, you will be surprised at how effective it is in a conditioning program. Within a relatively short time you will be able to increase both the rate and distance involved in your walking program. And most people are surprised to learn that adding a twenty-minute walk each day to their usual activity can result in a weight loss of a pound a month, an impressive twelve pounds each year! (Incidentally, there is absolutely no evidence that moderate exercise increases the appetite. Be assured that you can both exercise and lose weight effectively.) Although the 75 percent of maximum heart rate may not be achieved during these activities when they are incorporated into one's daily activities, over the long run these activities have a considerable positive conditioning effect.

THE METABOLIC COST OF ACTIVITIES

Many other activities of daily life can also be used for exercise conditioning, since all activities have a specific cost in terms of the amount of work they demand of the heart. To provide a quantitative measure of exertional activity, tables have been devised that relate various activities in terms of their usual metabolic cost. These tables use the convenient measurement called the MET, defined as the amount of oxygen used at absolute rest. Thus all activities can be described in multiples of METS, desk work using one to two METS while digging ditches uses seven or eight METS.

Table 10-1 gives the approximate metabolic costs of a variety of occupational and recreational activities. These data, published in a report sponsored by the American Heart Association, can be used in a number of ways. If you have determined that walking three miles per hour raises your heart rate to the 75 percent of maximum required for conditioning, you will see that cycling at six miles per hour or cleaning the windows are equivalent activities. These tables can also be used to roughly determine levels of activity that might cause symptoms in patients with angina. If an activity such as tennis doubles (four to five METS, for example) causes distress, the patient can then predict that ping-pong, with the same metabolic cost, may also precipitate angina.

CONDITIONING, INFORMAL AND UNSEEN

The second painless means of exercise is to enjoy sports activities. Here the key word is "enjoy," because the tense executive does himself no good at all when he repairs to the golf course or handball court to elevate his blood pressure further in an all-out effort to win. Competition in games is necessary in professional sports, but the pressured and possibly coronary-prone individual must learn to slow down and enjoy his leisure.

If the drive to win is so great that it interferes with the release of tension built up in the course of daily living, competitive sports are definitely not the answer. Golf, tennis, and handball are all fine games if you relax at them. If the drive to win comes be-

TABLE 10-1

APPROXIMATE METABOLIC COST OF ACTIVITIES* (including resting metabolic needs)

	Occupational	Recreational
1½-2 METs† 4-7 ml O_2/min/kg 2-2½ kcal/min (70-kg person)	Desk work Auto driving‡ Typing Electric calculating machine operation	Standing Walking (strolling 1.6 km or 1 mile/hr) Flying,‡ motorcycling‡ Playing cards‡ Sewing, knitting
2-3 METs 7-11 ml O_2/min/kg 2½-4 kcal/min (70-kg person)	Auto repair Radio, TV repair Janitorial work Typing, manual Bartending	Level walking (3¼ km or 2 miles/hr) Level bicycling (8 km or 5 miles/hr) Riding lawn mower Billiards, bowling Skeet,‡ shuffleboard Woodworking (light) Powerboat driving‡ Golf (power cart) Canoeing (4 km or 2½ miles/hr) Horseback riding (walk) Playing piano and many musical instruments
3-4 METs 11-14 ml O_2/min/kg 4-5 kcal/min (70-kg person)	Brick laying, plastering Wheelbarrow (45-kg or 100-lb load) Machine assembly Trailer-truck in traffic Welding (moderate load) Cleaning windows	Walking (5 km or 3 miles/hr) Cycling (10 km or 6 miles/hr) Horseshoe pitching Volleyball (6-man noncompetitive) Golf (pulling bag cart) Archery Sailing (handling small boat) Fly fishing (standing with waders) Horseback (sitting to trot) Badminton (social doubles) Pushing light power mower Energetic musician

256

MET Level	Activities
4-5 METs 14-18 ml O_2/min/kg 5-6 kcal/min (70-kg person)	Painting, masonry Paperhanging Light carpentry	Walking (5½ km or 3½ miles/hr) Cycling (13 km or 8 miles/hr) Table tennis Golf (carrying clubs) Dancing (foxtrot) Badminton (singles) Tennis (doubles) Raking leaves Hoeing Many calisthenics
5-6 METs 18-21 ml O_2/min/kg 6-7 kcal/min (70-kg person)	Digging garden Shoveling light earth	Walking (6½ km or 4 miles/hr) Cycling (16 km or 10 miles/hr) Canoeing (6½ km or 4 miles/hr) Horseback ("posting" to trot) Stream fishing (walking in light current in waders) Ice or roller skating (15 km or 9 miles/hr)
6-7 METs 21-25 ml O_2/min/kg 7-8 kcal/min (70-kg person)	Shoveling 10/min (4½ kg or 10 lbs)	Walking (8 km or 5 miles/hr) Cycling (17½ km or 11 miles/hr) Badminton (competitive) Tennis (singles) Splitting wood Snow shoveling Hand lawn-mowing Folk (square) dancing Light downhill skiing Ski touring (4 km or 2½ miles/hr) (loose snow) Water skiing

TABLE 10-1 (continued)

	Occupational	Recreational
7-8 METs 25-28 ml O_2/min/kg 8-10 kcal/min (70-kg person)	Digging ditches Carrying 36 kg or 80 lbs. Sawing hardwood	Jogging (8 km or 5 miles/hr) Cycling (19 km or 12 miles/hr) Horseback (gallop) Vigorous downhill skiing Basketball Mountain climbing Ice hockey Canoeing (8 km or 5 miles/hr) Touch football Paddleball
8-9 METs 28-32 ml O_2/min/kg 10-11 kcal/min (70-kg person)	Shoveling 10/min (5½ kg or 14 lbs)	Running (9 km or 5½ miles/hr) Cycling (21 km or 13 miles/hr) Ski touring (6½ km or 4 miles/hr) (loose snow) Squash racquets (social) Handball (social) Fencing Basketball (vigorous)
10 plus METs 32 plus ml O_2/min/kg 11 plus kcal/min (70-kg person)	Shoveling 10/min (7½ kg or 16 lbs)	Running: 6 mph = 10 METs 7 mph = 11½ METs 8 mph = 13½ METs 9 mph = 15 METs 10 mph = 17 METs Ski touring (8+ km or 5+ miles/hr) (loose snow) Handball (competitive) Squash (competitive)

*From Fox, S.M., Naughton, J. and Gorman, P.A.: Physical Activity and Cardiovascular Health, **Modern Concepts of Cardiovascular Disease,** 51:21-30, 1972, with permission of the authors and the American Heart Association, Inc.

†1 MET is the energy expenditure at rest, equivalent to approximately 3.5 ml O_2/kg body weight/minute.

‡A major excess metabolic increase may occur due to excitement, anxiety, or impatience in some of these activities, and a physician must assess his patient's psychological reactivity.

258

tween you and your enjoyment, try swimming, walking, or any of the less demanding noncompetitive sports.

If you can handle team sports without killing yourself in the drive to win, you might see if your local Y or community center offers volleyball, basketball, or softball. Always be sure to warm up before and cool down after each game, and be certain that you gain more release than tension from playing for your team.

For most people over the age of thirty-five, individual sports activities usually provide more in the way of exercise and the desired relief of tension because they do not emphasize group pressure to perform and win. Swimming is an excellent means of conditioning, requiring only a Y or club membership for implementation. Again it is important that stamina and endurance be built up gradually over a period of time until you are able to swim a quarter- or half-mile regularly. Swimming improves muscle tone throughout the body, and because it is the most dynamic exercise it is excellent for conditioning the heart.

Bicycling is another pleasant and effective way to exercise. If you live in the suburbs, try doing your local errands on a bike; on the weekends a longer period of cycling about the neighborhood can be an interesting and pleasant diversion. As with any form of exertion, it is best to start with only short distances planned, keeping in mind that the distance you pedal going away from home must also be covered to return. Try to go out in the uphill direction so that you can return to your home on the downhill grade.

If you live in a rugged or hilly area, invest in a good geared bicycle and use the lowest gear most of the time until you have developed some stamina. The new adult-size tricycles are excellent for people who have not ridden a two-wheeled bicycle for many years. The effort and exertion needed to maintain balance on a two-wheeler are not needed on these "trikes," and because of this you can pedal more slowly, an important plus for individuals who are interested in conditioning.

Although skiing is a good solitary sport, it can lead to serious musculoskeletal or cardiac problems in the uninitiated or in those who attempt the sport when in poor condition. Adults over the age of forty who have never skied are probably well advised not to start.

Golf is an excellent semicompetitive sport that allows the

honest player to compete only with himself, seeking to improve his score rather than to "slaughter" the opposition. To increase the conditioning effect of golf, try not to use a cart or, if you do, park it some distance away to increase the walking you must do to complete the game.

Tennis is a marvelous game, much in the news today, that can be used by the sensible adult for exercise conditioning. Again the key is moderation: if you are out of condition or have not played in years, start with doubles and play for the exercise, not to win. Tennis is most effective played at least twice a week, not on consecutive days. This means that you will try to get in a game or two during the week rather than playing without letup over the weekend. If you are over the age of forty and have never played tennis, it is especially important that you approach the game gradually, if at all. Handball, squash, and paddle tennis are strenuous games and should be played only by those who are well conditioned by steady exercise.

Fishing and hunting can be used by really serious fans for conditioning by the simple expedient of adding as much walking as possible. Bowling, skating, and other individual activities can also be used in conditioning, as can gardening and other chores about the house. All have a certain metabolic cost and, when approached with a view toward increasing one's level of activity, can be used as part of an overall exercise program.

All of the exercise conditioning activities suggested here should be done regularly and relatively frequently. All fulfill the requirement of involving motion of the body and all are pleasant methods of increasing one's endurance and conditioning the heart and cardiovascular system.

Chapter 11

Sex and the
Human Heart

The answer to the question, "Is sex good for my heart?" is "Yes." For many reasons, not the least being the sheer joy of it, sex is—or should be—a restorative and beneficial human activity. The healthy, symptom-free adult can enjoy sex to his particular *maximum* (defined as what feels good and does best for him) without fear of damaging his heart or cardiovascular system. In terms of the heart, sexual activity provides an excellent release of tension that is physiologically untaxing. Moreover, it alleviates stress by way of an extremely pleasant form of activity, a substantial benefit in this age of anxiety and overuse of sedatives and tranquilizers.

STRESS AND ITS RELEASE

If stress is as important in the development of coronary heart disease as recent work seems to indicate, then its release by sexual or other nonchemical means must be considered an important health measure. As noted earlier, the individual's *response* to the stress of his daily life appears to determine its toll upon him. Stress seems to damage the human organism by its constant wear and tear on the system; the individual whose temperament continually causes him to call up his maximal emotional reserves is obviously reacting to the stress of daily life in a harmful and ultimately destructive way.

Since the amount of stress-caused damage depends on the individual's pattern of responses, anything that helps one to deal with life's anxieties and frustrations has to be considered healthful and beneficial. Unfortunately, many of the methods that man chooses to help him tolerate the stress of daily life are harmful and ineffective. Alcohol and other drugs, cigarettes, or the abuse of tranquilizing medication, for example, cannot be depended upon to really help in the lifelong struggle to cope with stress.

The psychological, mind-oriented means of handling stress are discussed in Chapter 6 and I repeat my belief that people can change their attitudes toward life and its problems in order to live a healthier and less stressful existence. But there are also at least two physical means that appear to help men and women cope with stress. One is regular physical exercise: "feeling good" after a tennis game or a round of golf is usually the result of release of tension. For this reason, regular exercise is highly recommended as one means of modifying the coronary risk factor of stress. The other even more effective physical means of handling stress is sexual activity; sexual satisfaction richly deserves its recognition as the best tranquilizer available.

Sex appears to work its wonders through a complex interplay of physiological events and psychological effects. In physiological terms sexual arousal begins with relaxation as the parasympathetic branch of the autonomic nervous system is turned on. If anything interferes with this relaxation phase—the male's preoccupation with business or other everyday problems, the female's lack of trust in her partner, or perhaps a mutual fear of discovery—sexual arousal becomes difficult to achieve.

As stimulation increases, the sympathetic nervous system comes into play. Pulse rate and respiratory rate begin to rise, culminating finally in the orgasm, which is primarily a response of the sympathetic nervous system. (The occasional involuntary ejaculation of semen which occurs without an erection in young men when they get nervous is a manifestation of the sympathetic nervous system that leads in this case to an inappropriate reaction.)

Following orgasm the sympathetic nervous system shuts off almost immediately, and with its release there is a feeling of deep calm that often results in an extremely relaxing, restorative sleep.

These periods of sleep can last for a few minutes or for the entire night; in either case they are remarkably refreshing.

SEXUAL TENSION AND ITS RELEASE

Although these physical aspects of sexual response are easily explained from what we know of the physiology of the human nervous system, the psychological effect of sexual tension and its release are less clearly understood. A great deal of what we do know is based on our observations of ourselves and others in a state of sexual deprivation. Sexual frustration causes most people, men and women alike, to behave as if they were one raw nerve; the smallest, most insignificant upset will elicit a magnified and totally inappropriate emotional response. The sexually deprived have no insight into their behavior, real or imagined; their sexual frustration may cause them to sleep poorly, to magnify small problems into very big ones, and to suffer many other effects of stress, frequently unnecessarily and inappropriately, leading to considerable wear and tear on the cardiovascular system.

The slang term for this state of sexual tension is probably as descriptive as any: sexually deprived and anxious people are "horny." What is usually not appreciated is that "horniness" is not just related to a heightened response to sexual stimulation but is really a state of extreme sensitivity to any stimulus: touch, scent, sound, sight, and especially emotional strain. "Horny" individuals may paradoxically lose interest in sex but remain depressed, unhappy, anxious, and stressed by almost everything else. When sexual tension is alleviated, their personality suddenly improves and problems formerly considered insurmountable are readily overcome.

PHYSICAL COST OF SEX

If sexual satisfaction can help so dramatically in alleviating stress, how much then is "good" for the human organism? Again no one can say for anyone else, but it is clear that most people enjoy sex to their particular maximum, whatever it is. During sexual intercourse there is a steady increase in the heart and respiratory rates as well as an elevation in blood pressure. These climax, appropriately, at orgasm, and then return to the normal resting level rather rapidly. The breathlessness of orgasm lasts for only a few seconds, usually marking a joyful and significant release of tension.

Most healthy individuals know their sexual limits, but since sexual activity is a form of physical exertion it has long been considered helpful to have some kind of measure of its actual cost to the heart. In this country, Dr. Louis Hellerstein and his colleagues investigated the metabolic cost of a variety of human activities, in-including sexual intercourse. A group of men, half of whom had suffered a heart attack, were monitored by means of portable electrocardiographic equipment throughout a two-day period. By correlating the ECG with the self-reported log of activities kept by each individual, Hellerstein was able to derive an idea of the relative cost of the many normal activities of any two-day period.

Hellerstein's work is important because it measured the effects of the various activities of middle-aged men under normal home and working conditions, rather than in the artificial climate of the laboratory. We know that the maximum heart rate achieved during an activity correlates well with the amount of oxygen required by the heart to perform that activity and is thus a good indirect measure of oxygen cost. The most striking finding was that for many of Hellerstein's subjects heart rates attained during usual activities at home or on the job were as *high or higher* than those reached during sexual intercourse. For some men, driving a car, playing catch with the children, or even eating dinner led to a heart rate rise that was higher than that associated with sexual intercourse. One patient, a hard-working lawyer, showed a heart rate response when he was walking into the courtroom, arguing with an associate, or taking a trip to the washroom that was well in excess of the rate he attained during sexual intercourse.

The Hellerstein research also indicated that the period of increased heart rate during intercourse lasts for a very short time, reaching its maximum around the time of orgasm. During the two minutes before or after orgasm the average rate was between 80 and 100 beats per minute. At the time of orgasm the rate was 90 to 144 per minute for approximately thirty to sixty seconds. These rates were less than 75 percent of the maximum predicted heart rate in most individuals.

Hellerstein's work affirms that the maximum heart rate achieved during intercourse usually occurs at the moment of orgasm. Lasting for only ten to fifteen seconds, this is almost always far less than the tolerable maximum that would be predicted for that individual as a result of exercise testing. These rather modest heart rates, occurring for the very limited period of orgasm, suggest that the cost of sexual activity in terms of the heart's use of oxygen is rather small.

SOURCES OF POSSIBLE SEXUAL STRESS

From Hellerstein's work and the observations of others we conclude that the physical activity of sex appears to make only moderate demands on the heart in the context of a secure and satisfying relationship. But there are several elements that may contribute adversely to the physical cost of sexual intercourse, within or outside of marriage. Position, oddly enough, is not one of these; several studies, again using portable ECG recording equipment, have shown that there is not much difference in the demands placed on the heart by the varying positions of sexual intercourse. While I do not dispute these findings, I must point out that most people experiment until they find the position or form of sexual activity that is most comfortable and satisfying to them.

One of the significant statements of the so-called sexual revolution of our time is that nothing that two adults do with mutual joy and satisfaction is bad. And any long-term relationship, married or otherwise, bestows the incalculable benefit of allowing men and women to explore their own sexual responses and those of their partner. In the course of a long-term relationship, most people find the emotional and physical support they require; the actual position of sexual intercourse appears to make little difference either in terms of its physical demands on the heart or in its "rightness."

Several other elements, however, in the physical setting do appear to have some importance. It is probably not a good idea to have intercourse immediately after a large meal. The digestion of food requires considerable blood supply to the gut, and the added demands of sexual activity on the heart at that time may lead to some distress.

Extremes of temperature may also militate against sexual activity. If it is very cold try cuddling for warmth only; if it is very hot the physical exertion of coitus may be distinctly increased.

Alcohol may also play a part in increasing the physical cost of sexual intercourse. Although many people use alcohol to relax, it actually increases the heart rate by dilating the vessels. If you are planning to have "one for the road" in a sexual setting, make it tea or weak coffee.

Everyone has heard of cases of sudden death occurring during intercourse—the well-known "death in the saddle"—and several researchers have attempted to learn more about this puzzling event. A group of Japanese researchers investigated the circumstances of more than 5,500 cases of sudden death occurring in their country. A small number (34 out of 5,559) died during the act of coitus. Thirty of these, however, took place outside of the home, mostly in hotel rooms and presumably outside of marriage. On further investigation, it appeared to pathologists studying post-mortem tissues that extramarital intercourse may have placed a higher demand on the heart than would relations between husband and wife.

In almost all instances of sudden death associated with sexual activity, the fatal event occurred to a middle-aged man, away from home, with a strange, new, and usually younger partner; in most cases death occurred late at night, after a heavy meal that had included excessive alcohol. Under these circumstances, because of the inherent stress and tension of this type of illicit sex, sexual intercourse can be a significant physical strain.

Tension in any setting stresses the human organism, and it may be that the sexual tension of a fearful liaison produces a greater strain than one would expect. But any long-term relationship, married or otherwise, does not usually carry with it the demand inherent in a "one-night stand."

In general terms, if one desires sex and is sexually aroused—if one feels well enough to enjoy the sex act—in the context of a secure and considerate long-term relationship sexual activity is not detrimental to the heart. The test, I suppose, for every man and woman is the ultimate effect of intercourse: if it provides feelings of satisfaction, joy, and release of tension it is good for you. If you suffer guilt, anxiety, or emotional upset as a result of your sexual activities, or if you experience actual physical distress, there is something wrong and you need to change either the emotional or environmental circumstances of your sexual outlets.

SEXUAL PROBLEMS

From my observations, there are a great many men who *think* they have sexual problems. When pressed for details of this often vague but disquieting feeling, most men reveal a concern with what they think are waning sexual powers or an inability to have a "good enough erection." The fact is that as men grow older they do not lose their sexual powers, but the pattern does *change* significantly. Most men require more stimulation as they grow older and, if this and other pattern changes are disregarded, what is a perfectly natural accomodation to age may be allowed to grow into a genuine, and often totally unnecessary, problem.

Thus, in most cases, the most important criterion is the honest desire for physical sex. This means that the individual is not participating because of pressure from his partner or because of a need to demonstrate some vague kind of "sexiness." (Although most of what I have said in the context of this chapter is true for both men and women, the matter of the desire for sex and the ability to perform seem to be mostly a problem for males.)

One important aspect of sexuality, not widely appreciated, that can lead to misunderstanding and a breakdown in sexual communications is the change in male sexual physiology. As women mature into their middle thirties and forties, they may become less inhibited, more easily aroused, and much more rapidly receptive. The converse may be true in men, but in neither case is this a universal truth. Although it has nothing to do with potency and little to do with desire, many men are terribly distressed to suddenly find themselves sexually unable to do as they wish, exactly when they wish. Even as they verbalize that they would like to have sex, after a certain age men are sometimes chagrined to discover that it takes a little longer to achieve an erection sufficient for entry. Sometimes they require the active help of their partner, and not all men know how to ask nor do all women know how to respond to this request. This may be all the more alarming because among young men little more than the thought of sexual intercourse is usually enough to trigger full readiness. And young women frequently require long periods of foreplay before they are ready and long periods of intercourse before they are satisfied.

It is not within the province of this book to explore the irony of this and many other of the relations between men and women. In the ideal society perhaps old men would marry young women, working them up slowly to their sexual peak in their thirties and forties and then die off to free those women to marry young men —who are at their peak somewhere around the age of eighteen or twenty. If there is some paradise where this is the practice, I do not know of it.

As men grow older, it is unreasonable to expect the immediate sexual response of youth. Sometimes it is necessary to have the active assistance of the female partner and I applaud with vigor the suggestions of the more explicit sex manuals in this regard. Whatever the basis, women seem to be less inhibited today about their role in the sex act. A sensitive woman realizes that her husband may need help, especially if he is physically or emotionally worn from the stress of his daily life.

To expect a middle-aged man to express his desires on command, so to speak, with an immediate erection is unfair and ultimately unrewarding; recriminations and guilt can lead to bitterness and far more serious problems for both members of the pair. Manual and oral stimulation are now advocated by the more realistic experts and many people find them less physically taxing and more dependably satisfying than other more traditional forms of sexual activity. These forms of stimulation also allow men and women to pursue active and interesting sexual activities well into their seventies and even beyond.

SEXUAL ADEQUACY

Sexual ability probably depends to a large extent on sexual confidence, and anything that threatens that confidence can be destructive. In physical terms, the rule of thumb derived from Hellerstein's work is helpful; if you can manage two flights of stairs without difficulty you should have no trouble with the exertion required by sexual intercourse. If you have the desire for sex you should be able to perform without difficulty but it is essential that you not let the *fear* of an inadequate performance inhibit your actual ability. (*Very* rarely is sexual impotence due to a physical problem and, if it persists, it should be checked by a physician.)

The physical components of sex are probably less than half the story, however. Far more potent and far less well understood are the various psychological aspects of sex. Despite the many sexual handbooks available today, people still manage to work themselves and their partners into dismal states of sexual distress through ignorance and lack of understanding.

One disturbing kind of sexual problem is the loss of sexual excitement during intercourse, more dramatic in the male since it is usually accompanied by a sudden loss of erection. When such an episode occurs, it is extremely important that both partners know that it is a normal event, having absolutely nothing to do with the imminent or permanent loss of sexual ability. It is frequently related to extraneous worries and has little or nothing to do with the sex act itself. If the female partner is understanding and nonpunishing, in many cases her tactile or verbal encouragement is all that is needed to resume sexual play. Most often a problem of this kind derives from the many cares and worries that every man brings into bed with him. When this is the case, often just talking out the problem supplies the emotional support that is needed.

The most important thing, of course, is to make no more of a temporary loss of potency than is warranted. The occasional, transient loss of sexual ability is usually unimportant, having no significance other than that which both partners place on it. Making more of such an occurrence than is justified can trigger a cycle of sexual stress that can affect subsequent ability, and I urge all sensible men and women to tread lightly in this sensitive area.

If a single unsuccessful sexual attempt is magnified out of all proportion, the hitherto comfortable bed can become a tense sexual battlefield; a "problem" can also provide the opportunity for an exceptionally meaningful experience in the sex lives of two mature people—how the problem is handled depends entirely on the partners.

SEXUAL NEEDS OF WOMEN

A great deal is now known about the sexual neeeds of women, the result of pioneering research by Masters and Johnson and others. In a mature and nonpunishing relationship it is possible for all women to express their sexual needs openly. Although female sexual response is not usually as overt as the male's, there is no ~~estion that sexual tension builds and must be relieved. Sex is

needed for good health by men and women alike, and both partners must work to create the environment where the other can
verbalize or otherwise make known his or her needs without fear
of being punished or rebuffed. This requires love and sensitivity
on the part of each, compliance on occasion even when not really
interested and, more important, forbearing ever to use sex as a
means of power or control.

Sensing the sexual needs of one's partner becomes an unconscious art in most long-standing relationships, with certain sub-
liminal clues being picked up by each of the pair when the other
is in need of sexual release. In many long-standing relationships
the man and woman begin to cycle together, tension building for
each at the same rate.

Many women achieve genuine sexual satisfaction without
having a clearly labeled orgasm. Although sexual research has
added much to our store of knowledge, the pursuit of "something
better" by women who do not have bell-ringing, siren-screaming
multiple orgasms of the type described in some current best sellers
has made for strong feelings of inadequacy for both men and
women. This is extremely unfortunate and totally unjustified. I
suggest again, strongly, that each individual determine his own
sexual maximum, heeding only his own joyful measure of meaningful satisfaction.

The effort that it takes to make sex joyful to both partners is
well worth the trouble, both for the physical rewards and for the
great psychological benefits to be derived from the alleviation of
stress. Sexual satisfaction, given and received, yields the great emotional lift of loving and being loved, of caring and being cared for,
of demonstrating the ability to be a complete man or woman and
to give unselfishly to someone you love. These emotional returns
of sex with love are the positive and healthful aspects of the man/
woman relationship—greatly to be desired and sought after and
treasured.

Chapter 12

Everything
Affects the Heart

As long as heart disease remains one of mankind's more prominent problems, research into its prevention and treatment will continue throughout the world. I doubt that a single cause—or cure—for coronary heart disease will ever be found and I also suspect that many of the links between heart disease and the known risk factors will never really be "proved." The evidence that elevated serum lipid levels predispose to heart disease, for example, will probably remain just that—strong statistical evidence —although there is no question that the association between the two is compelling.

Continued research, of course, is the only way to discern the many inborn and environmental factors that may link each individual to his own risk of heart disease. Research efforts on all fronts are laudable and should have the wholehearted support of all adults.

The popular fallout from heart and lung research—the often misleading tidbits that find their way into the daily newspapers— are quite another matter. My quarrel with most popular accounts is not that they are sensational (although they usually are), but that they are often misleading. The claims in the papers of new "cures" for heart disease or new links between heart attacks and other factors often derive from a germ of truth or hypothesis that is in the process of being worked upon. Hypotheses do not sell newspapers, however, and what most laymen see are headlines reflecting the most sensational, or most horrific, aspects of the work.

I will try to discuss in detail all of the currently "hot" topics with regard to the heart, but more sensational claims will continue to appear in the pages of the daily newspapers. What is important is that you read the stories—not just the headlines—carefully. I have tried to provide enough background knowledge of the workings of the heart to enable you to make at least a preliminary evaluation of any sensational material that appears. If you have doubts or desire further information, you should ask your physician. His primary interest, always, is to improve the health of his patients; if there is anything new and efficacious in the treatment of disease he will know about it, and he is best able to relate it to your particular needs.

"HARD" AND "SOFT" WATER AND CARDIOVASCULAR DISEASE

In 1957 a Japanese researcher studying a curious difference in the incidence of strokes in various parts of Japan found that there was a significant correlation between the quality of the local water and the occurrence of cerebrovascular accidents. He noted that the ratio of sulfate to bicarbonate in the local river water used for drinking had a definite relation to the chance of the local inhabitants suffering a stroke. People living in areas of hard water supply had fewer strokes when compared to the inhabitants of soft water areas.

This demonstration that local geophysical properties of the environment might play a part in the etiology of vascular disease led investigators throughout the world to attempt to refute or support this conclusion and to determine whether other cardiovascular diseases could be correlated with the type of water supplied to an area.

Since that time many studies have been conducted in the United States and throughout the world. In virtually all of the studies an inverse relationship between the incidence of death from cardiovascular disease—especially atherosclerosis—and the hardness of the local drinking water was found; that is, the harder the water, the less cardiovascular disease in the area.

Water hardness is determined by the amount of mineral salts

in solution in the water. All water, except distilled water and rain-water which is actually distilled, comes in contact with soil, rocks, and organic matter. In these materials which make up the earth there are many substances including mineral salts that are soluble in water and, depending on the constituents of the environment, these substances go into solution in the local drinking water. The varied concentration of these minerals causes water in different areas to taste different.

The hardness of water is measured in parts per million, with very hard water containing more than 300 parts per million and very soft water less than 50 parts per million; that is, 50 molecules or ions of minerals per million molecules of water. Alternately, water hardness is measured by the concentration of calcium it contains, calcium usually being the most prominent mineral in solution in "nonsalt" water.

One of the typical studies, conducted in sixty-one boroughs in England and Wales, each with a population of over eighty thousand, showed that the incidence of deaths from cardiovascular disease was inversely proportional to the hardness of the water. Death rates ranged from about 700 to 860 per 100,000 population in towns with soft water to less than 550 per 100,000 people in areas with very hard water. Similar results were found in the United States; correlation of the death rates from arteriosclerotic heart disease per state and the degree of average water hardness in the state was highly significant negatively, with a higher incidence of cardiac deaths in the area where the water was softest. The incidence of deaths from hypertensive heart disease showed a similar relationship, being significantly higher in areas of soft water.

Change in cardiovascular mortality was also studied in a number of cities which changed the hardness of their water supply. In those that removed mineral salts to make their water softer the incidence of cardiovascular deaths increased significantly in the years after the water had been softened. In those American cities that increased the hardness of their water by adding minerals, the incidence of deaths due to cardiovascular disease decreased or increased to an extent that was significantly smaller than in those cities where the water had been softened.

Prediction calculations have suggested that over a twelve-year period the incidence of death from arteriosclerotic heart disease is 14 percent higher in areas of soft water than in hard water areas. Comparison of people matched for age, socioeconomic background, and sex in areas of very soft and very hard water showed that a slight increase in blood pressure, heart rate, and cholesterol levels occurred in the soft water areas. Whether these small increases were sufficient to explain mortality differences in the two areas remains unclear.

Analysis of the water supply with respect to a large number of elements (magnesium, silicon, bicarbonate and sulfate, calcium, vanadium, barium, copper, strontium, lithium, manganese—among others), demonstrates that no specific mineral, other than those usually related to water hardness, appears to play a role. There was, however, a weak suggestion that a higher level of copper and manganese might be directly related to an increase in the incidence of arteriosclerotic heart disease in soft water areas.

The correlation data on the hardness of local water and heart disease are not easily explained, but several theories have arisen. It has been suggested that it is either the absence of something needed in soft water that leads to arteriosclerotic heart disease or the presence of something in hard water that protects against its occurrence.

In Finland, the death rates from ischemic heart disease in areas of the country with soft water are nearly twice those of areas with hard water. Finnish researchers have suggested that the high soil content of magnesium found in the areas of low death rates may underlie the argument that hard water protects against heart disease. Since very low levels of magnesium are occasionally associated with the development of cardiac arrhythmias and may be implicated in sudden cardiac deaths, this is an intriguing hypothesis.

In both Scotland and Canada, researchers pursuing this lead have found lower magnesium levels in the heart muscles of subjects dying of myocardial infarction than in those dying of other causes. What remains to be proved, however, is whether the lowered level of magnesium in soft water areas actually plays a causal role in increased deaths from heart-related illness.

It should be emphasized, moreover, that the minerals present in hard water are all present in the food we eat in sufficient quantity and in high concentrations even in soft water areas, so it is unlikely that their absence in the water could lead to a deficiency. Elements positively correlated with heart disease (copper and manganese) that appear to be in higher quantities in some areas with soft water are also readily available in food so again it is unlikely that the overabundance of these elements in soft water areas is the answer.

Another interesting hypothesis has been suggested by a group of Canadian investigators. They confirmed that the incidence of cardiovascular deaths was significantly lower in areas of Ontario with hard water than in those with soft water. They noted, however, that the incidence of sudden death was also inversely correlated with water hardness. Ionized calcium is high in hard water; since low serum calcium occasionally plays a role in the initiation of abnormal cardiac rhythm disturbances—rhythm disturbances being the usual mechanism for sudden cardiac death—these Canadian researchers postulated that the slightly higher intake of ionized calcium in hard water areas is the protective mechanism present in hard water. (It is partly because of the hard water data that food faddists have rather simplemindedly suggested high calcium supplements as a preventive for heart disease. There is no evidence that calcium supplementation has any effect whatever on the development of heart disease.)

Although the calcium ions in hard water may be more available to the body than the calcium in food, the large intake of calcium in the normal diet casts some doubt on the theory that calcium exerts some protective influence. A more significant effect may be the corrosiveness of soft water. Hard water is slightly alkaline, whereas soft water is acid. The slight acidity of soft water causes it to slowly corrode metal pipes and to leach small amounts of metals out of the pipes and into the water.

Among the minerals leached into the water are important amounts of cadmium, antimony, and lead; each in only a few parts per million. The leaching out occurs when water stands in pipes for long periods of time when the faucets are closed and the water is not flowing. These metals are not present in any meaningful amounts in the source of the water supply but are added by the pipes within buildings. Laboratory work has shown that cadmium, lead, and antimony are concentrated in the kidneys and liver, and when these minerals are given to experimental animals hypertension results. It has also been reported that a high content of cadmium is found in the urine of hypertensive humans.

All of these mechanisms for the well-documented relationship of water hardness to cardiovascular deaths remain as yet hypothetical; further investigation and more developed theories will most assuredly be forthcoming in the future. At this time it is not justified to start popping calcium supplements; it may be wise, however, for those who live in soft water areas to consider running the water for a few minutes every morning before drinking or using it for the morning coffee. In this way the water that has been standing in metal pipes overnight and which may contain increased amounts of cadmium and antimony will be flushed away. It may also be wise not to soften drinking water, either in the home or community water supply.

COFFEE DRINKING

In 1972 the Boston Collaborative Drug Surveillance Program reported that among hospitalized patients diagnosed as having a myocardial infarction (heart attack), the frequency of heavy coffee drinking was approximately twice that of patients who were in the hospital with other diagnoses. These data were derived from questionaires that were filled out prior to discharge by every medically able patient admitted to the twenty-four cooperating hospitals in the Boston area. Patients were asked about drugs, alcohol, coffee, tea, cigarettes, and a variety of other substances taken either chronically or intermittently to determine the communitywide use of over- and under-the-counter medications and any possible relationship of their use to various illnesses.

When the diagnosis of myocardial infarction was correlated with the habitual intake of either none, one to six, or more than six cups of coffee per day, the Boston investigators found heavy coffee drinkers more than twice as prevalent among heart attack patients than among controls (patients admitted with other diagnoses); the prevalence of moderate coffee drinkers was about one and one-half times as great. No comparable increase in tea drinkers was found; the same percentage of patients drank large amounts of tea in both the myocardial infarction and control groups.

Other studies, both before and after their publication, have not agreed with the Boston findings. In the Framingham study, where five hundred initially healthy individuals were followed for approximately twenty years, there was only a weak correlation between heart attacks and coffee drinking that was not statistically significant. In three other studies (one sponsored by the National Research Council, another an epidemiological study of Western Electric employees, and the third by the Kaiser Permanente Clinic, a large health maintenance organization) either a weak correlation or no relationship was found.

Various theories have been put forth to reconcile this disparity. First, the percentage of heavy coffee drinkers among the controls in the Boston study was smaller than in any of the other studies. Approximately 20 percent of the controls in other studies were heavy coffee drinkers, as compared to the 9 or 10 percent in the Boston study. This suggests that the control population in the Boston study, possibly because they were sick enough to be hospitalized with other illness, probably did not drink as much coffee as normal people would.

Second, not all patients who had myocardial infarctions were included in the study. Only those who survived to be brought to the hospital and then lived and were well enough to be polled a few days after admission could be included. Since we know that more than 50 percent of the people stricken with myocardial infarction die before reaching the hospital and that another 15 to 20 percent die during the first two days of hospitalization, the Boston study may actually have selected out only those patients who tolerated their heart attacks. This could lead one to wonder whether coffee may actually have exerted a protective effect on those surviving a myocardial infarction, a highly unlikely hypothesis.

Third, heavy coffee intake correlates with other characteristics in the population. Many people with "coronary" type of personalities are heavy coffee drinkers. They tend to be heavy smokers as well. This latter factor has been invoked to explain the slight propensity to myocardial infarction in studies other than the Boston Drug Surveillance Program.

The mechanism of a possible relationship between coffee and myocardial infarction remains unclear. It is tempting to consider the high intake of caffeine as causative. Caffeine has an effect similar to sympathetic nervous stimulation, causing rises in blood pressure, heart rate, and strength of contraction of the heart—all of which increase the heart's need for oxygen—as well as generally increasing wakefulness and nervousness that also increase the work of the heart. Moreover, caffeine is a cardiac irritant and can stimulate the heart to have extra beats and sudden episodes of very rapid heart action. Tea drinking, however, which also has a high caffeine content does not correlate in any study with the occurrence of myocardial infarction.

Another possible mechanism that has been postulated concerns the effect of coffee on blood clotting. If a clot forms inappropriately in a blood vessel it is normally broken up after a time by substances in the bloodstream called *fibrinolysins*. These fibrinolysins are inhibited by substances found in coffee other than caffeine, and theoretically such small clots would not be removed as rapidly. (It is interesting that tea does not inhibit the action of the fibrinolysins.) In theory, the persistence of such clots might make the individual more prone to the development of myocardial infarction.

It has also been suggested that the high intake of sugar and of milk or cream with coffee drinking might play a role, but several of the studies mentioned above looked into this aspect and discarded it as untenable.

In view of the conflicting data, what is the best course to follow? Again, this is a situation where a possible risk factor—not yet "proved" or completely understood—can be modified by a slight change in one's living habits. Although the exact role of coffee drinking is not yet proved, one can advance sound reasons for moderation. If you are not a coffee drinker, do not become one. If you drink more than six cups a day, cut down to no more than three. If you can, try switching to tea or possibly decaffeinated coffee for at least some of your coffee breaks.

Caffeine is a known stimulant and if you notice any kind of abnormality in heart rhythm or if you are troubled by nervousness or difficulties in sleeping, it is a good idea to cut out all beverages containing caffeine such as coffee, tea, and most of the cola-type soft drinks. The evidence indicting coffee is not yet strong enough to warrant removing it from your life altogether; moderation, however, is always a good idea.

VITAMINS AND HEART DISEASE

Everyone would like to find a neat, simple, cheap, safe, and easy way to control his environment, his health, and his fate. Some turn to religion, others to superstition or astrology. Many who might be expected to have more good sense follow the food faddist, the natural food enthusiast or the vitamin buff. Now none of these is intrinsically harmful but, when food faddism is pushed to the extreme and this concern dominates all others, there is a good chance that one's health might suffer.

The problem is that there is always someone ready to take advantage of the unwary, who can figure the angles and exploit ignorance or human need to his own benefit. In recent years we have seen the growth of a number of pseudonutritionists, some with impressive but questionable credentials, who tout various vitamin and mineral preparations for the relief of everything from impotence and falling hair to cancer. Very often people who are in need of genuine medical care fall for this mumbo jumbo and neglect conditions that might otherwise be easily handled by current medical means.

Most people are concerned with the health of their hearts, and they readily fall prey to the coronary disease quacks. Their usual method is to quote a medical researcher, inaccurately and out of context, to support the particular preparation they are selling. Even if their intent is sincere and honest, they often base their claims on anecdotal, testimonial, and spurious case histories. Very often their "cures" are real but the condition was never present in the first place; in other cases the claims are so outlandish as to defy any rational analysis.

The tip off, I think, is when the proponent of one or another miracle cure tells you with great emphasis how he is persecuted by "organized medicine." Medicine is not organized; every physician is free to advise his patients as he thinks best for their welfare and no physician would hesitate to try any treatment that has been tested and seems likely to help. Rather than withhold some marvelous new treatment, most doctors would rush to use it, assuring themselves and their cured patients a niche in the pantheon of medicine.

The fact is that every one of the vitamin-based treatment

methods has been subjected to careful laboratory scrutiny, and none has been found to possess the curative powers claimed for them by their advocates. Some may have a limited value in heart disease and, of course, where a real deficiency exists—highly unlikely in this and other well-fed countries—adding a vitamin supplement may be absolutely necessary. (Other than the rare condition of beriberi, there is no evidence that vitamin deficiency causes heart disease except when it is so severe that death is imminent.) There is nothing wrong with taking vitamins; the danger lies in neglecting all other methods of caring for your heart.

Vitamin E, vitamin C, and lecithin are currently receiving a great deal of attention in the popular press and in pseudoscientific magazines as cures for, or preventives of, heart disease. All are substances that have been known for many years, and because they do little harm—except when pushed to the exclusion of all other forms of treatment—they have received the serious consideration of many qualified researchers with interesting results.

VITAMIN E

In the late 1920s, laboratory workers noticed that animals fed sufficient calories and all the vitamins known to that time were sometimes unable to sustain pregnancy. Although they were able to live and function fairly well on the standard diet, laboratory rats who became pregnant aborted after about ten days and resorbed the fetuses. When grain oils were added to the animals' diet this inability to maintain pregnancy was reversed. Vitamins A, B, C, and D had already been named, so this new substance was dubbed vitamin E.

Chemical and separation analysis led to the isolation of a family of similar compounds that could replace the whole grain oils necessary for successful pregnancies in the laboratory rats. These compounds were named *tocopherols,* from the Greek word meaning to bear a child, and because they had the chemical characteristics of an alcohol. *Alpha-tocopherol* is the most active of the group nutritionally.

Research continued into the new vitamin substance and soon it appeared that animals rendered deficient in vitamin E over a long period of time by extensive artificial manipulation of their diet suffered widespread bodily effects, including testicular degeneration, liver cell death, brain damage, red blood cell destruction, bone marrow failure, and capillary breakdown. Each effect was seen in some species but not in others, although generalized muscle degeneration occurred after a long period of dietary vitamin E deficiency in several species. These animals would often show heart muscle degeneration; they would develop heart failure and die with dilated, fatty, weakened hearts.

All of these effects were seen only in animals whose diets were extremely deficient in vitamin E over long periods of time but, since vitamin E is abundant in fruits, vegetables, and in the "germ" part of whole grain, extensive dietary manipulation was required before any deficiency occurred. Research was continued to find a naturally occurring disease for which vitamin E could be considered treatment. Vitamin E was tried in women who suffered repeated miscarriages, in a wide variety of muscular and neurological disorders, and in a large number of other known disease states. Until 1947 all of these studies showed essentially no benefit to be derived from vitamin E.

In that year, a group of Canadian investigators headed by Dr. Wilfred Shute reported beneficial effects when vitamin E was used to treat heart disease of varying etiologies. They claimed good results in reversing some of the deterioration suffered by patients with hypertensive, coronary artery, and rheumatic heart disease. Since these are disease states with widely varying effects, medical researchers throughout the world attempted to replicate these studies in controlled research projects using large groups of patients. Unfortunately, studies conducted at Cornell, Duke, and Boston Universities failed to confirm the exciting reports of the Shute group. Under carefully controlled conditions, vitamin E was shown to have no more benefit in the treatment of heart disease than sugar tablets.

These findings that there is no therapeutic value in vitamin E were confirmed by similar studies throughout the intervening years. And yet in just the same way that people tend to remember only the good things about people who have died, the food faddists ignore the negative reports and continue to cite the original unsubstantiated findings, now almost thirty years old.

Research into other aspects of vitamin E continues, however, with some interesting results. Vitamin E works as an antioxidant, preserving essential body substances from "rust" or inappropriate chemical breakdown. The most important finding, perhaps, is that vitamin E is ubiquitous, present in almost all of the vegetable or grain foods that we eat. And the relatively small amount of vitamin E needed by the human organism makes it virtually impossible to find a genuine state of naturally occurring deficiency other than in patients with very severe malabsorption from their gastrointestinal tract. To date no one has found any form of heart disease that can be alleviated by supplementary vitamin E.

The most recent large-scale effort to identify a role for vitamin E took place in 1973 when an international symposium was held under the auspices of the agricultural grain industry. (The main surce of vitamin E is the oil derived from wheat germ.) Reputable nutritionists and researchers attending this conference reported three situations in which vitamin E appeared to have some possible value.

One group found vitamin E effective in decreasing the pain of intermittent claudication, a chronic cramping in the calves of the legs caused by narrowing of the major blood vessels. In similar studies, however, other workers found once again that the vitamin was no better than a placebo in the treatment of intermittent claudication. They pointed to the fact that the natural course of the disease varies widely—the pain being intermittent in nature.

The apparently beneficial effects of the drug in one study may have reflected only the tendency of the disease to subside when activity is increased or when the patient feels he should improve, that is, the placebo effect.

Another group studied the value of vitamin E in animals who were fed large amounts of unsaturated fats. As noted earlier, the presence of unsaturated fat appears to protect against the development of high cholesterol levels, but these substances are easily oxidized because of the double bonds in their chemical structure. In order to preserve the integrity of unsaturated fat and to keep them from being destroyed, animals on this diet appeared to require more vitamin E than those on diets containing reduced amounts of unsaturated fat.

Unsaturated fat, most often of vegetable origin, is always accompanied in nature by the tocopherols; thus when they are ingested in normal circumstances the amount of vitamin E needed to maintain their integrity is assured. When grains containing unsaturated fats are refined for the modern diet, the vitamin E may be destroyed and the extra amount of the vitamin that is needed to preserve the unsaturated fat may not be supplied. Again, however, the possible deleterious effect of the circumstance is not clear and may actually have little importance in the maintenance of human health.

The antioxidant effect of vitamin E has also been suggested as a possible aid in decreasing the damage caused by air pollution. Polluted air contains a number of oxides of nitrogen and sulphur that are potent oxidizing agents and much of the iritation and damage attributed to impure air may be due to this chemical action. Because of its effect as an antioxidant, vitamin E may prevent this damage.

In experimental animals the amount of vitamin E necessary to maintain health increases when the animals are exposed to impure and polluted air for long periods of time. The significance of this finding with respect to heart disease or to the effects of pollution on human health remains unclear at this time.

Although these three reports suggested avenues for continued research, all of the possible roles for vitamin E remain unproved and largely conjectural.

In recent years the possible effect of vitamin E on blood coagulation has received considerable interest. Initial reports that tocopherols reduce the tendency of the blood to clot have not been supported by subsequent studies. Along with a group at the Bronx Veterans Administration Hospital I recently investigated the action of vitamin E on platelet function, and we reported that it appears to have no effect on the tendency of platelets to aggregate and form clots. I must conclude, with others, that as yet no scientifically acceptable data show that vitamin E has any effect in the prevention or treatment of any form of heart disease in humans.

One investigator, Dr. Mac Horwitt, has reviewed the data concerning any beneficial effects of vitamin E and feels strongly enough to state that its use enriches only the sewers of this country, any vitamin E not needed by the body being excreted rather promptly. Since there is no evidence that vitamin E is harmful to the human organism, my position is that if the individual derives some comfort from taking the substance and can afford the money that it costs, then I do not insist that it not be taken.

VITAMIN C

In the current wave of interest in therapeutic uses of vitamin supplements, vitamin C has received attention as a possible anti-atherosclerotic agent. Again scientific support is sparse although there are some interesting data concerning vitamin C and its relation to the metabolism of cholesterol.

One of the problems with studies of vitamin C is that most of the laboratory animals traditionally used in research do not require the vitamin in their diets. Monkeys, rats, dogs, and mice all have the ability to manufacture the vitamin C that they need within their bodies. Guinea pigs, however, like man, do require an exogenous source of vitamin C and an interesting study reported in *Science* in 1973 makes use of this fact.

A Czechoslovakian investigator, Emil Ginter, bred a colony of guinea pigs who were deficient in vitamin C. He then injected radioactively labeled cholesterol and observed its rate of excretion or breakdown. (Cholesterol is excreted mainly by conversion to bile salts in the liver. The bile salts are secreted with the bile into the intestinal tract where they aid in the absorption of ingested fats and give the stool its characteristic color.)

In this study, the animals which were deficient in vitamin C were found to convert cholesterol to bile salts at a slower rate than normal controls. The result was an elevation of the level of cholesterol in the blood and in the liver. This study shows only that vitamin C deficiency can be a cause of faulty removal of cholesterol and its buildup in the bloodstream of guinea pigs. It is not yet clear to what degree this is important in humans and whether this finding has any significant effect on the development of atherosclerosis.

Other studies have suggested that high doses of vitamin C can prevent the appearance of atherosclerotic lesions of the aorta in animals maintained for a long time on highly atherogenic diets. The levels of cholesterol in the liver and in the blood serum were elevated in both the vitamin C and control animals but atherosclerotic lesions in the aorta were found to be significantly less frequent in animals whose diets included large amount of vitamin

C. This suggests a possible protective effect of vitamin C but again I must point out that animals do not naturally develop atherosclerosis at all unless fed a markedly distorted diet, in this case one extremely high in fats. For this reason the relationship of these and other findings to the "natural" occurrence of atherosclerosis in man remains unclear.

To date, studies in humans attempting to pin down the effect of vitamin C on serum cholesterol levels have been contradictory. In a study conducted in England, volunteers received one gram of vitamin C daily for a six-week period and cholesterol levels were compared with those measured for the six-week period preceding the study. At the end of the study the figures were analyzed with the following results. Volunteers under the age of twenty-five showed a trend toward lowering of cholesterol levels; there was little change in those twenty-five to forty-five years old; levels tended to increase in volunteers over the age of forty-five; and, in those with a history of atherosclerosis, there was a significant rise in blood cholesterol levels.

This is a strange mixture of results and Dr. Constance Spittle, who conducted the study, interpreted the latter findings to mean that the cholesterol measured in the blood of older patients was being mobilized from atherosclerotic lesions within the blood vessels. In her view the higher serum levels of cholesterol suggested that vitamin C was acting to reverse the atherosclerotic process.

There are reports that contradict these findings. In this country, B. Sokoloff reported that the level of blood cholesterol did not change in patients with atherosclerosis, although triglycerides decreased during administration of vitamin C. In a group of young men eighteen to twenty-four years of age, who were taking vitamin C in a study of cold prevention, the decrease in cholesterol reported to occur in the young English volunteers was not confirmed. In fact, subjects taking vitamin C had a significantly higher level of blood cholesterol than nontreated controls.

Thus the increase in blood cholesterol levels reported by Dr. Spittle may not be due to the breakdown of atherosclerotic plaque at all, but may actually reflect the enhanced production of cholesterol within the body. A rise of this kind in serum cholesterol levels is certainly undesirable, and it has been suggested that, until the mechanism for this effect is elucidated, older patients and those with known atherosclerosis would be wise to avoid high doses of vitamin C taken for any purpose.

Vitamin C has also been suggested as useful in the treatment or prevention of heart disease for other reasons. It is important in maintaining the vigor of ground substance and collagen, the materials that compose the connective tissue of the body. Prolonged vitamin C deficiency causes scurvy— a disease common among eighteenth-century sailors but rarely seen today—that is manifested by a breakdown in the connective tissue of the blood vessels that causes bleeding gums and a tendency to bruise easily. Some researchers have hypothesized that deterioration of the connective tissue in arteriosclerosis may in this way predispose blood vessels to the development of plaque, but this is highly theoretical and no evidence exists that such an effect actually occurs.

Vitamin C, also known as ascorbic acid, is an antioxidant and acts to maintain the integrity of body constituents. Like vitamin E, however, it is not known whether this antioxidant effect is of any clinical importance, although in theory it may have a bearing on the metabolism of body lipids such as cholesterol and triglyceride. Again there is no hard evidence that vitamin C will affect the development of atherosclerosis in humans and no data from a controlled trial have appeared to suggest that vitamin C can be of benefit in the treatment or prevention of heart disease in human beings.

LECITHIN

Lecithin is a lipid or fat that is found in vegetable oils and in the many foods that contain cholesterol, such as egg yolk. Along with cholesterol, lecithin is part of the lipoprotein complex within the body that serves to transport triglycerides in the bloodstream from the liver to the body's cells. Because lecithin acts to increase the solubility of the complex it has been suggested that as a dietary supplement it might keep cholesterol in solution in the blood, in this way helping to avoid its deposition in atherosclerotic plaques in the arterial walls.

Again the evidence in unclear. Lecithin is primarily an unsaturated fat, and we know that a diet rich in unsaturated fat tends to lower blood cholesterol levels. But there are no data to suggest that lecithin is different from any of the other unsaturated fats present in vegetable oils, and no studies to date have shown that lecithin has any significant effect in removing or preventing the deposition of cholesterol into the tissues or on arterial walls.

Like vitamin E and vitamin C, lecithin may be an antioxidant and may in theory have some beneficial effect for that reason. Again, however, there is little documented evidence to support lecithin either as a preventive or as a treatment for atherosclerosis or heart disease.

OTHER VITAMINS

From time to time there are reports in the lay press or in professional journals suggesting other substances as possible aids in the management and prevention of atherosclerosis. In recent years I have seen articles concerning the efficacy and possible value of pyridoxine and other B vitamins as well as reports on the use of minerals such as copper, manganese, and chromium. To date I know of no definitive study that proves the efficacy of any of these substances.

This does not mean that one must forget entirely about vitamin supplements and their possible uses. Considering all the claims made for various substances, and noting the sparse supporting data, I believe that a rational adult who is concerned with his heart and cardiovascular system should follow a prudent course. This means eating a balanced diet with generous amounts of fruits, vegetables, whole grain cereals, and whole grain breads. All of the substances discussed in this chapter—vitamin E, vitamin C, and lecithin—are supplied by a balanced diet of this kind. As people grow older, it is also probably a good idea to increase one's intake of bulk and roughage, in this way easing elimination.

You will, of course, try to lower your intake of cholesterol and saturated fats, replacing them wherever possible with unsaturated fats according to the principles set forth in Chapter 6. And, although it is probably unnecessary in most instances, a multivitamin tablet taken once daily will supply any nutrients missing from your diet. If you take a daily vitamin pill that makes you feel better, you are probably satisfying little more than your need to feel that you are doing something.

Any supplemental vitamin not needed by the body is excreted fairly promptly so if a subclinical deficiency state is present this moderate regimen will take care of it with no problem. What may be hazardous, however, is the disturbing trend toward huge doses, the so-called "megavitamin" approach. Excess in any form is usually bad and unless you are being treated by a physician for a specific problem, I see no reason for large doses of one or another vitamin or mineral.

In conclusion, after many years of interest and considerable research effort, the value of large doses of any of the known vitamins or minerals in the treatment or prevention of heart disease remains unproved and conjectural.

HIGH-FIBER DIET

Considerable attention has recently been focused on a high-fiber diet as a panacea that is good for everything. In regard to heart disease, it has been suggested that a high-fiber diet will reduce blood cholesterol levels. Although there is a possible rationale for this that involves the bile salts, the means by which the body excretes cholesterol, there are as yet only sparse scientific data supporting this claim, and one report refuting it was presented at the 1976 American Heart Association National Meeting.

There is, however, another good, though somewhat old-fashioned, reason for including roughage in the diets of people with coronary heart disease. One of the normal activities of living that may require considerable exertion is the elimination of stool. If constipation is present, straining at stool or bearing down to defecate requires what is essentially a Valsalva maneuver. This is a form of exertion that results in a sudden rise in blood pressure followed by a sudden drop. Strain of this kind also triggers a fast firing of the parasympathetic nervous system that slows the heart and in this way may precipitate an arrhythmia.

As a result of these many effects, some patients have anginal symptoms when they are at stool. For several reasons, then, a high-fiber diet which includes raw fruits and vegetables, whole grain cereals, and fibrous foods of all kinds may indirectly benefit someone with heart disease.

ALCOHOL

The first tranquilizing drug known to man, alcohol, has been alternately attacked as the bane of mankind or defended as the nectar of the gods that enables man to tolerate the injustice and frustrations of life. Called by some the wrecker of families and of careers, alcohol has also been considered the oil that lubricates and smooths many of the traumatic, awkward, and potentially unpleasant social situations and interrelationships among people.

Alcohol's effect on the psyche and disposition of mankind will forever remain controversial since what appears to make one person convivial and charming can turn another into an addicted and antisocial monster. Because of alcohol's importance to society and the pervasive extent of its consumption, government and private organizations have poured enormous sums of money into research concerning alcohol use and abuse. (Anyone who recognizes that he has a problem with drinking can write to the National Institute on Alcohol Abuse and Alcoholism, Box 2045, Rockville, Maryland, 20852, for information on programs designed to help him and his family; also he can call Alcoholics Anonymous, listed in the white pages of the telephone book.)

But we know that any drug that works affects the body in many ways, and alcohol is a drug with a wide range of actions. In the last twenty years research into the effects of alcohol on the heart have been especially productive. It is helpful to consider the results of alcohol use in those who have heart disease and in those whose hearts are normal; and to divide its effects into those which are due to acute alcohol consumption and those which are due to chronic usage.

Using this construct, investigators have looked at the acute effect of alcohol in doses equivalent to two or three shots of whiskey. In normal individuals, alcohol in this moderate amount led to relaxation of the vascular bed, an increase in the heart rate, and an increase in the amount of blood pumped by the heart per minute. These vasodilating effects were observed to occur in normal individuals with no change in blood pressure.

The vasodilating effect of alcohol has been recognized for years as being responsible for the "glow" produced by one or two drinks, with the relaxation of the peripheral blood vessels causing a measurable flush and feeling of warmth. In the normal individual this modest amount of drinking does not appear to depress the action of the heart; twelve ounces of Scotch, however, taken at one time, have been observed to have a mild but significant depressant effect even on normal hearts.

In subjects with coronary artery disease, however, alcohol use is not so benign. Three or four shots have been observed to cause a progressive decrease in blood pressure, a decrease in the amount of blood pumped by the heart per minute, a decrease in the amount of work the heart can do, and even changes on the electrocardiogram. There is little if any relaxation of the vascular bed and the heart rate response is lessened or absent altogether, suggesting that alcohol exerts a significant depressant effect on the hearts of people with coronary artery disease.

To explain this varied action, researchers have postulated that the acute effects of alcohol are twofold, direct, and indirect. Alcohol's direct effect is a general depression of the heart's ability to pump; its indirect effect is related to stimulation of adrenalin secretion. In the normal heart, the adrenalin effect masks or minimizes the depressing effect; the adrenalin stimulates the heart to greater function, in this way counteracting the negative and depressing effects. In patients with underlying heart disease, however, the direct effect predominates, partly because the heart is more sensitive to any depressant and partly because the heart's ability to respond to the adrenalin release is less marked. The net effect in patients with cardiovascular impairment is to further inhibit the heart's function. The greater the amount of alcohol ingested the greater the depressant effect, so high doses appear to affect even normal individuals by depressing cardiac function.

Does this mean that patients with coronary disease should not drink at all? Not necessarily. In moderation the relaxing effects of a small amount of alcohol may be of considerable value to the individual, so most physicians do not insist that coronary patients abstain completely from social drinking. In fact, a recent study correlating alcohol intake with risk of developing coronary disease in Japanese men living in Hawaii found that the risk of coronary events *decreased* among moderate drinkers as compared to teetotalers. The source of alcohol was beer in most instances with those drinking up to forty ounces a day having a lesser incidence of coronary disease than nondrinkers. The incidence of coronary problems was 45.6/1000 in nondrinkers, 25.9/1000 in consumers of ten or more ounces of beer a day. The reasons for these findings remain conjectural. The recent finding that high density lipoprotein levels in the blood tend to be elevated by moderate alcohol intake may play a role; high density lipoprotein levels are significantly correlated with a lesser incidence of coronary disease possibly because HDL may act to remove cholesterol from vessel walls. It is however, also likely that the anti-stress effect of alcohol plays a role in this beneficial effect. What must be emphasized, however, is that more than one or two drinks may have some important adverse effects and along with most physicians I suggest that coronary patients avoid excessive alcohol intake.

People with a long history of alcoholism, rather than developing a tolerance for alcohol, appear to become more sensitive to its depressive effects on cardiovascular function. Individuals who drink heavily and have no evidence of underlying heart disease appear to respond even to small amounts of alcohol in a manner that is similar to the impaired response of those with abnormal hearts.

The chronic ingestion of large amounts of alcohol has long been known to be associated with heart disease. A significant number of alcoholics develop severe heart failure, with marked enlargement of the heart, shortness of breath, swollen ankles, decrease in exercise tolerance, disturbances in heart rhythm, and, on occasion, sudden death. Chronic alcoholics with hearts that appear normal often show abnormalities of heart function when tested with advanced equipment, and the response of the heart to exercise is almost always impaired.

Alcohol in large quantities for long periods of time clearly damages the heart. Alcoholic heart disease (or alcoholic myocardiopathy), characterized by symptoms of heart failure, was long thought to be caused by the poor nutrition that is often associated with chronic alcoholism, especially a deficiency of thiamine and other B vitamins. It was subsequently shown, however, that myocardiopathy occurs in alcoholics who remain well nourished and that in the large majority of cases therapeutic doses of vitamin B have no effect.

Alcoholic heart disease is now thought to be due to a direct toxic effect of alcohol on the heart muscle itself; in some way the alcohol interferes with metabolism within the individual cells of the heart muscle. Changes in enzyme levels, the same kind of "leakage" that occurs during a heart attack, as well as changes in the metabolic function of the heart have been shown to occur in experimental animals fed alcohol over a long period of time and in alcoholic patients studied intensively.

There are some investigators who feel that alcoholic heart disease may be caused by some substance found in wine, spirits, and beer. (One local epidemic in Canada some years ago was traced to cobalt salts added to beer to increase the size of its "head"; needless to say, cobalt is no longer used in the brewing process.) And there are other studies that suggest that the mechanism by which alcohol damages the heart is related to its effects on the body's ability to fight viral and bacterial infections. According to this view alcoholic myocardiopathy may actually be the end stage of a viral inflammation of the heart to which alcoholics are prone by virtue of their lowered resistance to infection.

Although there are few data to suggest that alcohol has any causal effect on the development of coronary disease, chronic alcoholism is known to increase the blood levels of lipids such as cholesterol and triglycerides. What is not yet known, however, is whether this situation actually leads to excessive arteriosclerotic deposition. As if all this were not enough, chronic alcohol ingestion is also associated with liver disease, problems with the nervous system involving both the brain and peripheral nerves, premature senility, impotence, ulcers, gastritis, gastrointestinal bleeding, bronchitis, pneumonia, and tuberculosis among other unpleasant events. As the body ages it loses some of its tolerance for alcohol, so the same amount of liquor that you could handle with no trouble in your forties may cause a problem after the age of fifty.

In summary, then, small amounts of alcohol do not appear to have a significant effect on the normal heart. In patients with underlying or overt coronary disease, however, or in chronic alcoholics, even moderate amounts of alcohol can depress the heart's function; excess amounts can cause serious and acute cardiovascular events. My advice, then, succinctly put, is moderation: use only enough of this potent drug to achieve a mild and transient tranquilizing effect.

DRUG ABUSE AND THE HEART

I do not think a book of this kind written twenty years ago would have discussed the possible effects on the adult heart of heroin, barbiturates, cocaine, amphetamines, and other mood-altering "recreational" drugs. In those halcyon days drug abuse was limited to a rather small number of people, usually young and on the fringes of the law, and its role in the development of heart disease did not seem to warrant a great deal of investigation.

During the last ten years or so there has been a wide increase in the amount, variety, and extent of drugs used: more people appear to be taking more drugs over a longer period of time. Since research into the cardiovascular effects of improper drug use is just beginning, all we know so far is that the usual drugs of abuse produce a wide range of social, psychological, and physical consequences. Research into illicit drug use has already produced evidence of direct and harmful bodily effects. These are powerful pharmacologic substances that in most investigations have been shown to have adverse effects on the heart.

HEROIN

Heroin is a manufactured derivative of opium. After it is injected into the bloodstream, it changes into morphine and has the same physiologic effect as that valuable medicine. In proper doses, heroin, like morphine, can be effective in relieving the pain of a heart attack or the acute shortness of breath associated with severe heart failure or pulmonary edema; in England heroin is used by physicians as a sedative and pain reliever.

But like morphine, in the larger doses associated with nonmedical use, heroin has a marked depressant effect on the respiration and can cause the breathing to stop. Through its extensive effects on the autonomic nervous system heroin can cause the heart to slow down and stop, can lower the blood pressure precipitously and can lead to sudden death.

Tolerance to heroin or morphine builds up quickly and physical addiction can occur fairly rapidly. If either drug in the addicted individual is stopped abruptly, the autonomic nervous system can go haywire, producing a cacophony of life-threatening effects on the heart rate and blood pressure in addition to the well-known "cold turkey" distress involving the gastrointestinal tract and other organ systems. The stress of sudden withdrawal on the heart can be lethal.

In addicts who have been withdrawn from heroin the tolerance to the dose goes down markedly, and a shot of the same amount they were using while addicted may cause respiratory arrest, circulatory collapse, or shock and sudden death.

These effects are inherent in the pharmacology of heroin and morphine and must be considered a certain result of their use. Illicit heroin and its preparation carry with them a whole new set of lethal possibilities. The heroin available on the street is almost always cut with other substances. Quinine is often used because its taste on the tongue seems to suggest a more potent dose. But quinine taken in the veins in large enough doses can stop the heart abruptly, or it can lead to rhythm disturbances or a possibly lethal drop in blood pressure.

Other fillers may cause similar damaging effects in the cardiovascular system. If they are not soluble but remain as particles their injection can lead to scarring in the vessels of the lungs or other parts of the vascular system. An extensive destructive inflammation of the blood vessel walls known as *necrotizing vasculitis* that is often seen in heavy drug users may be due to the heroin itself or to the filler.

The most common effect of heroin on the heart occurs frequently in both addicts and in nonaddicted people, the so-called "users" who take the drug only on occasion. This complication is related to the unsterile conditions in which the drug is taken and the bacteria frequently injected along with it. These germs can form bacterial colonies on the valve structures of the heart and destroy them. The patient is severely ill, with high fever, and then finally goes into heart failure as the valves begin to develop large leaks. Although bacterial endocarditis is also occasionally seen in patients with valve abnormalities due to rheumatic fever, the endocarditis associated with illicit drug use is usually more severe and more often fatal.

Endocarditis of this type can occur in any situation where substances are injected into the veins in unsterile conditions. A most disquieting form of drug abuse involves crushing drugs that come in pill form, putting them into a solution of some kind, and injecting them. This use of illicit drugs also carries a high risk of infection to the heart valves. Moreover, the talcum powder that is usually used as a filler in drugs or capsules can lead to serious reactions in the lung vessels when taken intravenously.

AMPHETAMINES

The amphetamine group of drugs, including methedrine, or "speed," Ritalin, and a few others, are potent sympathomimetics; that is, they produce strong sympathetic nervous system stimulation that is similar to a large shot of adrenalin. The precipitous rise in blood pressure, the marked increase in heart rate, and the increase in the strength of contraction of the heart caused by these drugs place a severe strain on the heart and increase its need for oxygen. If any coronary disease is present, amphetamine use can cause severe angina and may precipitate a heart attack.

The stimulatory effects of these drugs on cardiac function, even in people with apparently normal hearts, can precipitate the development of severe rhythm disturbances, and the sharp rise in blood pressure that occurs after these drugs are taken can cause strokes. Overdoses of amphetamine-type drugs first stimulate the cardiovascular system but after a time cause it to fatigue and collapse, with death usually caused by shock, lowered heart rate, and respiratory arrest. Like adrenalin, amphetamines and other sympathomimetics may also cause blood to clot more rapidly and may play a role in the inappropriate and dangerous formation of clots within the blood vessels.

Amphetamines were widely used in the past to aid in weight reduction or in the treatment of depression, but we know much more now about their hazards and strong potential for addiction. Their use is now strictly controlled, as it should be, and anyone who takes these drugs for any nonmedical reason really needs to have his brains examined.

COCAINE

Cocaine is a drug that is occasionally used as a local anesthetic. This is its *only* safe use. When "snorted" or injected intravenously it can be lethal. Cocaine's effects are similar to those of the amphetamines except that early in its action the rise in blood pressure may cause a paradoxical reflex slowing of the heart rate. As its action proceeds in the body, cocaine can cause the heart rate to speed up inordinately, producing serious—sometimes lethal—rhythm disturbances and sudden death.

Addiction to either cocaine or the amphetamines can develop

rapidly. Withdrawal effects on the heart are often severe and can lead to death. Although some tolerance to the excitatory effect of drugs may occur, the propensity and sensitivity to rhythm abnormalities does not diminish. Increasing the dose to achieve the same high is dangerous and can lead to sudden cardiac death.

BARBITURATES

Barbiturates in the usual prescribed doses have little effect on the cardiovascular system other than a mild drop in blood pressure. The major changes occur with either overdosage or addiction.

Large doses of barbiturates depress the body's respiratory center, causing breathing to slow and possibly stop. At high dosages the blood pressure may drop to dangerously low levels and shock and death can occur. The effects of barbiturates on respiration add to the depressant effects of any drugs such as tranquilizers or alcohol that may also be present, and the combination may make an even previously tolerated dose lethal. (The widely publicized deaths of certain public figures were reported to have been caused by the deadly combination of alcohol and barbiturate sleeping pills.)

Barbiturates are physically addicting; this means that the body will undergo severe physiological withdrawal symptoms when the drug is stopped abruptly. Following a long period of addiction withdrawal is fraught with danger as hyperexcitement and hyperactivation of the cardiovascular and central nervous systems replace the barbiturate effects, often with resulting convulsions or death. People who are addicted to barbiturates should *never* attempt to treat themselves by abruptly stopping the drug ("cold turkey" method). Detoxification must *always* be done under close medical supervision.

HALLUCINOGENS

Hallucinogenic agents such as LSD and mescaline have not been studied extensively, but they appear to affect the cardiovascular system by increasing the heart rate and mildly raising the blood pressure. The use of these drugs, however, is especially hazardous to the cardiac patient because the response they elicit is severe and unpredictable, often producing an emotionally disturbing and sometimes persistent anxiety state. Along with this dysphoric reaction there is frequently a marked sympathetic nervous system response with a rapid heart rate and an increase in blood pressure that may put a serious strain on the heart.

Documented cases of sudden death occurring as a result of glue sniffing or aerosol inhalation are usually due to serious heart rhythm disturbances. These agents may also affect the blood cell production centers in the bone marrow. The frequent tragedies of sudden collapse and death seen in teenagers who inhale model airplane glue for its hallucinogenic effect is thought to be caused by the occurrence of fatal cardiac rhythm disturbances.

MARIJUANA

My guess is that marijuana is the most used of all the so-called "recreational" drugs. Because of the widespread interest in its possible decriminalization marijuana is also the most studied of the drugs of abuse, although a great many questions remain to be answered about the consequences of its regular social use. Everyone is most anxious to learn more about marijuana, but we must remember that it took more than forty years to determine the hazards of tobacco smoking and to take the first tentative steps toward its control in the United States and abroad.

The effect of marijuana on the cardiovascular system has been shown to be related in large measure to stimulation of the sympathetic nervous system, with a resultant increase in heart rate and a mild increase in blood pressure. This effect appears to be related to the dose, with higher doses producing greater rate increases. As with the hallucinogens, the stimulating effect of marijuana also appears to be related to the user's emotional response to the drug. Electrocardiographic changes and rhythm disturbance have also been reported after marijuana use.

The drug can also have a significant effect on breathing. The more potent forms of marijuana and various types of hashish have not been studied specifically, but their physiologic effects would be expected to be greater because the active ingredient in each is thought to be the same (delta-9-tetrahydrocannabinol or THC), varying only in the quantity contained.

In patients with coronary artery disease and angina, marijuana is definitely contraindicated. Exercise tolerance—the amount of work that can be done before anginal chest pain occurs—decreases markedly after smoking even one marijuana cigarette. This pain is thought to result from an increase in the heart's need for oxygen caused by the sympathetic nervous stimulation of the drug.

CHRONIC MISUSE OF VALUABLE DRUGS

Three valuable drugs used in the treatment of cardiovascular disease have been abused from time to time, often with dire consequences: digitalis and diuretics in the name of weight reduction, and amyl nitrate for some vaguely defined sexual "high."

Until fairly recently, digitalis was used by some few people as an anorexiant, or appetite-curber, to help in weight reduction. Unfortunately, the dose needed to curb the appetite is very high and at the toxic level. At the toxic level, digitalis frequently produces heart rhythm disturbances that are extremely dangerous. In the past digitalis was sometimes prescribed along with thyroid hormone and amphetamines to achieve rapid weight loss. The resulting stimulation—increased heart rate and blood pressure, speeded-up metabolism, sleeplessness, and agitation—acts to increase the work of the heart, producing a serious strain and a tendency to possible fatal rhythm disturbances.

Digitalis remains a safe and useful drug when properly administered to cardiac patients and monitored by a physician, but it should never be used for any purpose without medical supervision.

Much the same is true of diuretics. For years dieters popped a diuretic pill and basked in the glow of an immediate two- to four-pound weight loss. Although the scale may have shown it, there was no actual weight loss at all, for the water and salt lost as a result of diuretic action was immediately replaced by a body far wiser than its thirsty owner.

Repeated use of these drugs to keep the weight down is dangerous. With the loss of large amounts of water and salt, the potassium level in the blood can go down to dangerously low levels; in addition the blood can become too alkaline. Symptoms of tiredness, weakness, and muscle cramps can develop and, after prolonged inappropriate use, serious cardiac rhythm disturbances can be precipitated.

Diuretics are safe and excellent drugs when they are used properly for the appropriate medical indication. They can lead to discomfort and trouble—and have no beneficial effect whatever over the long term—when they are used for weight reduction.

Amyl nitrate was one of the first forms of the nitrate class of compounds used for the treatment of angina pectoris. It has been largely superseded by sublingual nitroglycerine that is now the main drug used for the relief of acute angina.

Amyl nitrate comes in a small, thin glass "pearl" that is covered with gauze. When used to relieve angina, the glass bulb is crushed and the fumes of the drug are inhaled. Amyl nitrate works in the same way as nitroglycerine by relaxing the arteries and veins, decreasing both resistance to the ejection of blood from the heart and the amount of blood returning to the heart—in this way decreasing the size of the heart. Decreasing the peripheral resistance and decreasing the size of the heart reduce the heart's need for oxygen, and in this way angina is relieved. As with morphine, there may also be a dilatation of the coronary arteries and an increase in blood flow and oxygen available to the heart muscle.

Amyl nitrate is not widely used for the treatment of angina because of two properties of the drug. The first is that the dose of nitrate is absorbed too rapidly and in many patients can cause an excessively marked drop in blood pressure that is followed by a reflex marked increase in blood pressure and heart rate within minutes of its use. Both the marked decrease in blood pressure and the reflex sharp rise in blood pressure and heart rate may make the angina worse. The drop in blood pressure may lead to a significant decrease in coronary flow and the reflex rise in blood pressure and heart rate will increase the heart's need for oxygen. The second reason is that any beneficial effect of amyl nitrate is relatively short-lived.

Amyl nitrate has been abused by a segment of one of our subcultures because sniffing it is purported to increase the pleasurable sensations that occur with sexual orgasm. It is not clear why amyl nitrate should have this effect but most probably it is related to the hypotension (low blood pressure) associated with the sudden inhalation of the drug. This drop in blood pressure may lead to a decrease in the supply of blood and oxygen to the brain. A lack of oxygen to the brain can produce a form of euphoria similar to that experienced by aviators in nonpressurized cabins at high altitudes just before they pass out.

If amyl nitrate is used for the relief of angina, the patient should not stand up abruptly for several minutes after inhalation because the blood pressure is low and dizziness may result.

I hate to be stuffy about it, but I fail to see any pleasure at all in amyl nitrate inhalation. The drug smells like vomit and its inappropriate use can be hazardous—with fainting, brain damage, and possibly death among its consequences, especially if the dose is increased. (No fatalities following abuse of amyl nitrate in this context have been reported, but it is unlikely that witnesses would acknowledge this as a possible cause of death.)

In summary, I find little good to say about any of the currently abused "recreational" drugs. Most are related to psychosocial deterioration of one kind or another and all are associated with particular stresses to the heart and cardiovascular system. For anyone over the age of thirty-five and most particularly for anyone with a history of heart disease, their use is most foolhardy.

My own feeling is that *all* drugs should be taken only for specific conditions, under the supervision of a physician, and only for as long as is needed to clear that condition. If you have no medical need for drugs, be grateful and do not look for trouble.

Chapter 13

The Symptoms of Coronary Artery Disease: When to Seek Medical Help

The primary purpose of this volume has been the prevention of coronary artery disease. To that end the normal and abnormal working of the heart has been discussed and the concepts currently felt to be operant in the etiology of coronary disease have been presented in detail in an effort to emphasize the important role of the known risk factors in the development of the disease. Methods to control these risk factors have been discussed at length with the hope that the reader will use these techniques for decreasing his risk of the development of coronary disease.

It is important, however, to include in any treatise on prevention of coronary heart disease information on the recognition of early signs of the disease. This is especially important in coronary disease due to a number of factors. Firstly, over 50 percent of those who suffer a heart attack die before they reach medical attention. Of those who make it into a hospital with an adequately staffed and equipped coronary care unit only about 10 to 20 percent die. All of the advances in therapy of heart attack that have been developed over the past fifteen years are sadly of no benefit to those who did not recognize that they were in trouble early enough to get the proper help. Coupled with this well-documented observation, it has been recently shown that up to 75 percent of patients who make it to a coronary care unit with a heart attack,

301

have had symptoms suggestive of coronary disease for months or weeks before they sustained the actual heart attack. Whether prompt early care might have prevented the event in each individual case remains uncertain, of course, but possibly in many, the heart attack might have been postponed or its deleterious effects might have been lessened. It is not known how many of those who die before reaching a hospital might have been helped; but by extrapolating the figures it is likely that many lives might have been saved, had early warning signs been heeded.

Coronary artery disease presents clinically in one of two ways, either as angina or as a heart attack. Prior to a clear-cut heart attack there are frequently vague symptoms suggestive of angina.

THE SYMPTOMS OF ANGINA

Angina pectoris (the literal meaning in Latin is pain in the chest), is the term used for the pain caused by ischemia of the heart muscle. If a coronary artery is sufficiently narrowed, with its diameter decreased by greater than 50 percent, the ability to increase blood flow through the artery is compromised. At rest there may be enough blood flow to satisfy the needs of the heart muscle dependent on that artery. With greater physical exertion or with the emotions of fear or anger, an increase in heart rate, blood pressure, and strength of contraction of the heart results because of the outpouring of adrenalin. The narrowed artery is unable to allow the increase in blood flow that is necessary to fulfill the new need for more blood and oxygen. The heart muscle that is deprived of the needed blood flow becomes ischemic and it sends signals to the brain that are interpreted as pain in the chest, the left shoulder, the upper arm, the left neck, the left side of the jaw, the left elbow, or a number of other areas. Continuation of the activity that caused the heart to require more blood flow or any increase in that activity will cause the pain to become more severe. Stopping the activity and relaxing will cause the need for augmented blood flow to abate, the heart will decrease its added activity and after a short period of time the ischemia will be relieved and the discomfort will disappear. The more severe the coronary disease, the less the exertion necessary to precipitate the symptoms.

The hallmark of the determination of whether a pain is due to ischemia of a portion of the heart muscle, i.e., due to angina, is this relationship between the discomfort and activities or events that cause the heart to require more blood flow. Any discomfort that occurs between the ear lobes and umbilicus (belly button) that is brought on by exertion and relieved by rest can be angina. Common precipitating causes are rushing to catch a train or bus, running up more flights of stairs than is customary for the individual, walking rapidly uphill, walking in the wind or on a cold day, carrying any heavy object such as a suitcase, a bag of groceries or a set of golf clubs, pushing or pulling a heavy object or participating vigorously in competitive sports. In some patients angina occurs only when they are angry or in a verbal or physical fight. Others have angina only if they exercise after a heavy meal; the meal alone or the activity without a meal may or may not precipitate the angina. Occasionally sexual intercourse will be the only activity that causes angina. Any type of exertion, physical or emotional, can cause angina.

Typically angina is not described as a pain but rather as a feeling of heaviness or squeezing in the chest with radiation to the left shoulder or the left arm. Angina is frequently atypical however, and may feel like an ache in these areas or as if something were not swallowed properly and has left a "lump in the throat." Pain in the jaw, sufficiently severe to send the patient to the dentist, or shoulder pain suggestive of arthritis or bursitis, without any discomfort in the chest, is occasionally the major complaint. Indigestion with either a burning sensation or a feeling that it is necessary to belch is commonly a sign of angina. Angina may actually be relieved by belching in some patients. Some patients may have pain only in the elbow, skipping the shoulder and chest, or discomfort only in the left wrist. The discomfort in the chest is usually central, over the lower or upper part of the breast bone. It is only rarely associated with pain in the nipple area. It may present as a tight band across the entire chest, involving not just the left side; and may involve both arms or just the right arm rather than the typical involvement of the left arm and shoulder. Typically, the pain of angina is not relieved by antacids, whereas the heart burn pain due to overeating or reflux of acid from the stomach up the esophagus (the swallowing tube) usually is relieved.

Because the pain of angina is frequently so atypical it is wise to see a physician if you have any form of discomfort in the upper part of the body that is brought on by exertion and relieved by rest. It is more indicative of angina if the discomfort is associated with shortness of breath, dizziness or a cold sweat. By questioning the patient closely, checking a resting ECG, and, in some instances, performing a stress test, in most instances it can be readily determined whether or not the symptom is angina.

The Symptoms of Heart Attack

The pain of impending or early heart attack is similar to the pain of angina but instead of being precipitated by a relatively extraordinary exertion it is either precipitated by an activity that was tolerated without discomfort a few hours or a few days previously or occurs at rest. Moreover, it is usually more severe than angina and almost always lasts longer than fifteen minutes. In some instances it may abate with complete relaxation but then recurs with any further activity or development of emotion. It is very frequently associated with a feeling of marked weakness or the sense of impending doom that many patients who have had a heart attack speak of later. The patient often breaks out in a cold sweat and may feel dizzy, and on occasion he may faint. Associated with the discomfort there is usually a sudden loss of appetite, if eating, and nausea is common. Frequently the patient will vomit, either spontaneously or by inducing it himself in an effort to make himself feel better. Some patients have a sudden urge to defecate or urinate. Palpitations, a sense of extra beats, skipped beats, or an unpleasant fluttering in the chest, will occasionally accompany the discomfort. In some instances the heart attack victim will want to sit still because any activity increases the discomfort, whereas in others there is a marked restlessness and the patient will walk around to try to walk off the pain. Because of the subtle breathlessness that frequently occurs with a heart attack, many patients complain of a feeling that the room has become stuffy and they either walk out for "fresh air" or open a window.

The pain associated with a heart attack is usually more typical than is angina, and more severe. A heavy strong aching sensation in the center of the chest with pain also in the left arm and shoulder is the most common presentation. Patients describe the pain as if "an elephant were sitting on my chest," as if "a vise were being tightened across the chest," as if there were a "constricting band across the chest," as if a "bubble" or a "balloon" in the chest were "getting bigger and bigger and were about to burst." In other instances, the pain has a distribution and quality similar to that described for the more atypical presentations of angina. The hallmark that distinguishes the discomfort of myocardial infarction from that of angina is the fact that the pain lasts longer, is more intense, is precipated by an activity that was previously tolerated, or occurs at rest and is usually associated with other symptoms such as shortness of breath, sweating, dizziness, nausea, and a feeling that something is seriously wrong.

Frequently people who are with a heart attack victim sense that something serious is happening even before the patient complains of discomfort. The patients are usually pale and may be ashen grey, or appear as if all the blood had drained from their face. There may be a sheen of sweat over the forehead and bridge of the nose. He may have a look of concentration as if he just thought of something important. Occasionally there is a dramatic clutching of the chest or the patient may pass out, but this is relatively unusual. In most instances the patient will stop what he is doing and will either leave the room to go to the bathroom or to go out "for some air." When asked, the patient will usually volunteer that he feels funny with a sense of indigestion and fullness in his chest. If the observer has training and can feel the pulse he may find it inappropriately rapid (greater than 90) or inappropriately slow (less than 60) and he may feel it to be irregular with extra beats and/or skipped beats. Frequently, however, the pulse is normal.

Understanding what is happening physiologically during a heart attack makes the symptoms less mysterious, though not less frightening. If an area of a coronary artery is suddenly occluded totally, the area of heart muscle fed by that artery will undergo changes. With the lack of oxygen associated with blockage of coronary blood flow the muscle becomes ischemic, and as in angina, signals are sent to the brain that are sensed as discomfort in the chest, the left shoulder and other areas as described for angina. With angina, however, the lack of blood flow and oxygen is only a relative one, because the blood flow is not completely stopped but is inadequate for the increased needs of the heart for oxygen that has been caused by the activity that precipitated the angina.

The discomfort will cause the victim to stop his activity and bring the system back into balance, with whatever blood flow that is possible through the narrowed coronary, again becoming sufficient for the now decreased needs of the heart muscle. With total occlusion of the blood vessel, the area dependent on the coronary arteries flow is starved even if the victim is at rest and the heart is beating quietly. For this reason the pain does not go away but lasts even if the patient is at complete rest, and for this reason frequently the pain occurs when the patient is completely relaxed.

Shortly after complete cessation of coronary blood flow, the area of the heart fed by the blocked coronary artery stops contracting. The pain may continue unabated or may let up a bit, but rarely does it go away entirely. With a part of the heart not contracting, cardiac function is compromised, the output of the heart suddenly is decreased and the symptoms of dizziness, not feeling right, and shortness of breath may develop. As a response to this decrease in heart function, and also as a response to the pain, the sympathetic nervous system is triggered and an outpouring of adrenalin and other catecholamines occurs. This causes the skin vessels to constrict and the ashen grey appearance; it causes the feeling of nervousness and restlessness; and it may cause the heart to beat faster or to have extra beats or skipped beats. The cold sweat is also a sympathetic nervous system response.

The parasympathetic nervous system is also stimulated by the pain and decrease in cardiac output. The nausea, urge to defecate or urinate, and an inappropriate slow rate are the effects of the parasympathetic stimulation. Fainting that is occasionally seen with the onset of a heart attack can be a parasympathetic response due to the slow heart rate or due to a reflex drop in the blood pressure. It may also be caused by the loss of cardiac output due to a very large area of heart muscle not functioning, or it may be due to a rhythm disturbance that is caused by electrical irritability of the ischemic area or by sympathetic nervous system stimulation.

Over hours after the onset of the occlusion, some collateral coronary blood vessels open up and deliver a small amount of blood from another coronary artery to the area of heart muscle fed by the occluded vessel. In the majority of patients this additional blood flow is not sufficient to keep alive all of the muscle at risk and over a period of time irreversible damage occurs to most of the ischemic heart muscle. The heart muscle cells die within a few hours and over the next three weeks or so the damaged muscle is replaced by scar tissue. In most instances, if the patient survives the first two days, he will survive the attack and though he has lost (forever) some of his functioning heart muscle, there is usually enough left for him to eventually resume a relatively normal life.

DEATH RELATED TO HEART ATTACK

At the first suggestion of a heart attack it is vitally important that a patient be taken to a hospital immediately. There are a number of reasons for this but the main one is that proper medical care may save his life. To appreciate this it is important to understand how patients die from a heart attack. There are basically three causes of death related to heart attack.

The first and most common mode of death out of a hospital is related to disturbances of the heart rhythm. An area of damage in the heart can serve as a focus to stimulate extra beats that are ineffective, cutting down on the amount of blood that the heart can pump. If these abnormal beats occur very frequently or in long runs, the heart is unable to supply the body with the blood flow it needs. More importantly, the decrease in pumping ability of the heart may further decrease the amount of blood delivered to the coronary arteries and the area of infarction or dead muscle will be enlarged. Extra beats of this sort may degenerate further into ventricular fibrillation, an arrhythmia that results in no effective heart beat; and, within a few minutes, if the rhythm is not normalized, the patient will be dead. The stimulation of the sympathetic nervous system that occurs at the time of a heart attack serves to facilitate the occurrence of these dangerous rhythm problems. The myocardial infarction may also involve areas of the heart that lead to very slow rhythms, either by causing heart block or by reflex. These slow rhythms may lead to cardiac standstill and death or may so compromise the amount of blood that can be pumped from the heart that coronary blood flow is affected and progression of cardiac damage as described above may occur.

The equipment in the coronary artery unit is specifically designed to monitor the patient's heart beat and warn of these serious rhythm problems; the staff of the coronary care unit is specifically trained to recognize, prevent, and treat these dangerous rhythms before they cause irreversible problems. Almost all of the increase in the survival after heart attack that has been effected in the past fifteen years because of the availability of coronary care units, has been through the management and prevention of these rhythm abnormalities. The sooner the patient gets to a coronary care unit or to where his rhythm can be constantly monitored the less is the chance that he will die of an arrhythmia associated with a heart attack.

The second cause of death is a mechanical one. With a heart attack, a portion of the heart muscle ceases to function and eventually is irreversibly lost. If more than 40 percent of the muscle of the left ventricle stops contracting, the heart is unable to pump sufficiently to supply the needs of the body for blood flow. The patient's blood pressure will drop or he may develop severe heart failure. Eventually the heart is unable to support life and the patient dies. To some extent the amount of heart that will be lost is predetermined at the time of the onset of the heart attack, but not entirely. By getting the patient to the hospital immediately, the amount of eventual damage may be decreased. Alleviation of pain, sedating the patient so that the heart has to work less, in some instances decreasing the blood pressure to normal levels if it is high, and in some instances, blocking the sympathetic nervous system may decrease the need of the heart for blood flow and of the compromised part of the heart muscle for oxygen. If there is less need for oxygen, the muscle cells on the periphery of the ischemic area may then receive sufficient oxygen from the small amount of blood that flows to the area by way of collateral vessels to keep them alive and the amount of heart muscle that will be lost will be less. In rare instances, mechanical pumps can be used to support the failing heart and surgery on the coronaries can be attempted.

The third cause of death associated with heart attacks involves the complications that occasionally occur after an attack. These include clots that originate in the legs, that go to the lungs, strokes, infections, pneumonia, or progression of the infarction. Complications may be prevented by early medical attention and can be treated promptly if they occur in the hospitalized patient.

There are other important reasons for bringing the possible heart attack victim to the hospital immediately. First, in many instances, the symptoms may not be due to a heart attack, but rather to indigestion, shoulder arthritis or bursitis, muscle spasm, or other benign causes. *This cannot be determined with assurance without appropriate medical evaluation,* that in most instances includes examination by a doctor and the recording of an electrocardiogram. In many instances, even with an ECG, the diagnosis cannot be made and the patient may have to be admitted and observed with repeated ECGs and blood tests to make sure that a heart attack has not occurred.

Secondly, the symptoms suggestive of a heart attack may not be caused by one, but may abate spontaneously, even though they have been due to a problem in the coronary arteries. The attack may be a serious warning. In recent years a syndrome (a set of symptoms and other findings) has been described that has all the symptoms of a heart attack but does not result in any heart damage. It has been shown that the majority of these patients have severe coronary artery disease and within a few years, many will either have a heart attack or die suddenly. Patients who present with this syndrome are usually followed closely by their doctors and are frequently studied with coronary arteriography. If sufficiently severe coronary lesions are found, these patients are commonly considered for coronary bypass surgery. By heeding the warning of this "intermediate syndrome" (intermediate between angina and heart attack) heart attack may be prevented and life possibly prolonged. The mechanism for this syndrome is not totally understood but may involve the occurrence of small clots that block an area of narrowing in a coronary artery and then break up spontaneously and the artery is unblocked. In other patients an area of coronary narrowing may suddenly spasm and close off, only to open again a few minutes later. Probably the most likely mechanism is that an artery is critically narrowed. With a subtle increase in oxygen need by the heart, sufficient flow is unable to get through the area and symptoms develop. With the decrease in the requirement for oxygen that occurs with the sedation and bed rest given to all patients with a possible myocardial infarction, the system is again in balance. Regardless of the mechanism, a patient who has come through an attack that might have been a heart attack should consider himself fortunate but he should also consider himself warned and should take heed by remaining under competent medical care.

I hope that utilization of the methods and principles of risk factor alleviation described in this volume will result in the reader never having to worry about these symptoms of active coronary disease. However, knowledge of the symptoms of angina and heart attack will forearm the individual so that he can best ensure that he has a long normal pleasant life by dealing promptly with any consequences of coronary disease if they occur.

Index